Get Through

PLAB Part 1: 500 Single Best Answer Questions

Get Through

PLAB Part 1:
500 Single Best Answer Questions

Una Coales
MD FRCS FRCS(ORL) DRCOG DFFP MRCGP
General Practitioner
London, UK

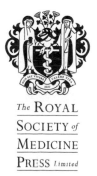

The ROYAL
SOCIETY of
MEDICINE
PRESS Limited

©2006 Royal Society of Medicine Ltd

Published by the Royal Society of Medicine Press Ltd
1 Wimpole Street, London W1G 0AE, UK
Tel: +44 (0)20 7290 2921
Fax: +44 (0)20 7290 2929
E-mail: publishing@rsmpress.co.uk

British Library Cataloguing in Publication Data
A catalogue record for this book is available from the British Library

ISBN: 1-85315-638-8

Distribution in Europe and Rest of the World:

Marston Book Services Ltd
PO Box 269
Abingdon
Oxon OX14 4YN, UK
Tel: +44 (0)1235 465500
Fax: +44 (0)1235 465555
Email: direct.order@marston.co.uk

Distribution in USA and Canada:

Royal Society of Medicine Press Ltd
c/o BookMasters Inc
30 Amberwood Parkway
Ashland, OH 44805, USA
Tel: +1 800 247 6553/+1 800 266 5564
Fax: +1 419 281 6883
Email: orders@bookmasters.com

Distribution in Australia and New Zealand:

Elsevier Australia
30–52 Smidmore Street
Marrikville NSW 2204, Australia
Tel: +61 2 9517 8999
Fax: +61 2 9517 2249
Email: service@elsevier.com.au

Typeset by Phoenix Photosetting, Chatham, Kent

Printed in the UK by Bell & Bain Ltd, Glasgow

Contents

Preface

I sat and passed PLAB in 1994, when the exam consisted of five modules: a negative marking MCQ paper, a written paper, slide identification, orals, and an English tape and essay. At that time, I had to pass all five modules in one sitting to clear PLAB or resit the entire exam again. Since then, thankfully, a series of changes have been made to the exam to make it more reasonable to pass. The latest change was made in September 2004, when single best answers were reintroduced to Part 1. PLAB Part 1 is now a 3-hour written exam consisting of 70% extended matching questions (EMQs) and 30% single best answer (SBA) questions. The exam contains 200 questions in total and may contain photographic material. In other words you have 54 seconds to answer each question! The good news is that there is no negative marking, so feel free to make an educated guess. Another piece of good news is that if you should fail Part 2, you do not have to resit Part 1; you still retain credit for clearing Part 1.

This book accompanies *PLAB: 1000 Extended Matching Questions* and contains 500 SBA questions reflecting both current medical practice and the current PLAB syllabus.

Una Coales
ufcmd@aol.com

I would like to dedicate this book to Dr John Coales (1815–1843), a family relative. He was born on Waterloo Day in 1815, won the first gold medal as the best medical student at Guy's Hospital in 1837, but sadly died of tuberculosis 6 years later.

Recommended Texts and References

American Psychiatric Association (2000) *Diagnostic and Statistical Manual of Mental Disorders*, 4th edn. American Psychiatric Association, Washington D.C.

Collier J., Longmore M. *et al.* (2006) *Oxford Handbook of Clinical Specialties*, 7th edn. Oxford University Press, Oxford.

Kasper D.L., Braunwald E., Fauci A., Hauser S., Longo D., Jameson J.L. (2004) *Harrison's Principles of Internal Medicine*, 16th edn. McGraw-Hill, New York.

Fitzpatrick T.B., Johnson R.A., Wolff K., Suurmond R. (2005) *Color Atlas and Synopsis of Clinical Dermatology*, 4th edn. McGraw-Hill, New York.

Harris M., Taylor G. (2003) *Medical Statistics Made Easy*, Taylor & Francis, London.

Longmore M., Wilkinson I., Rajagopalan S. (2004) *Oxford Handbook of Clinical Medicine*, 6th edn. Oxford University Press, Oxford.

Jawetz E. *et al.* (1989) *Review of Medical Microbiology*, 18th edn. Appleton & Lange, Connecticut.

Kumar P.J., Clark M. (2005) *Clinical Medicine*, 6th edn. Baillière Tindall, London.

Sinnatamby C., Last R.J. (1999) *Last's Anatomy Regional and Applied*, 10th edn. Churchill Livingstone, London.

Royal Pharmaceutical Society of Great Britain (2005) *British National Formulary*. British Medical Association, London.

Rubenstein D, Bradley J, Wayne D. (2002) *Lecture Notes on Clinical Medicine*, 6th edn. Blackwell Science Publications, Oxford.

Simon C., Everitt H., Kendrick T. (2005) *Oxford Handbook of General Practice*, 2nd edn. Oxford University Press, Oxford.

The Editorial Board (2004) *Advanced Life Support Course Provider Manual*, Resuscitation Council (UK), London.

The American College of Surgeons (2001) *Advanced Trauma Life Support Course for Physicians*, 7th edn. ACS, Chicago.

Tomb D.A. (1999) *Psychiatry*, 6th edn. Lippincott, Williams and Wilkins, Baltimore.

Unwin A., Jones K. *et al.* (1995) *Emergency Orthopaedics and Trauma*. Butterworth Heinemann Ltd., Oxford.

500 Single Best Answer Questions

1. A 59-year-old post-menopausal woman presents with a month of PV bleeding. On speculum exam, the cervix appears normal and there is no vaginal discharge.

   What is the SINGLE most *appropriate diagnostic* test?

   A. Cervical smear
   B. Hysteroscopy
   C. Pelvic ultrasound
   D. Serum FSH level
   E. Transvaginal ultrasound with endometrial sampling

2. A 24-year-old woman reports she has missed the first pill in her second pill pack. She had unprotected sexual intercourse (UPSI) 2 days ago.

   What is the SINGLE most *appropriate management*?

   A. Advise her to continue as usual as she had UPSI during her pill-free break
   B. Advise her to miss the next pill-free break before commencing pack 3
   C. Advise her to take the first and second pills now and continue as normal
   D. Fit an IUCD
   E. Prescribe levonorgestrel 1.5 mg stat

3. An 80-year-old woman is brought in by her family as they are concerned as she has been getting progressively more confused over the past few months. She is disoriented to time, place and person and often wanders the streets aimlessly.

   What is the SINGLE most *likely diagnosis*?

   A. Alzheimer's disease
   B. Delirium
   C. Parkinson's disease
   D. Subdural haematoma
   E. Vascular dementia

4. A 2-year-old boy is brought in by his parents as they are concerned as he has a past history of febrile convulsions. His last convulsion was 6 months ago. There is also a family history of epilepsy.

What is the SINGLE most *appropriate management*?

A. Arrange EEG
B. Arrange MRI
C. Arrange sleep studies
D. Commence regular lorazepam
E. Educate the parents on when and how to administer rectal diazepam

5. A 50-year-old man presents with right-sided hemiparesis. There is a bruit on neck auscultation.

What is the SINGLE most *appropriate investigation*?

A. Blood pressure measurement
B. Carotid doppler
C. CT scan of head
D. MRI scan
E. Slit-lamp examination

6. A 17-year-old presents to A&E with a traumatic limp. On exam, he has a foot drop and is unable to dorsiflex or evert his left ankle. Sensation is lost over the front and lateral side of the leg and dorsum of the foot.

What is the SINGLE most *likely diagnosis*?

A. Common peroneal nerve injury
B. Femoral nerve injury
C. Sciatic nerve injury
D. Superficial peroneal nerve injury
E. Tibial nerve injury

7. A 22-month-old girl has severe dehydration. You are unable to gain peripheral venous access.

What is the SINGLE most *appropriate management*?

A. Administer subcutaneous fluids
B. Arrange for a PEG
C. Insert a central line
D. Insert an NG tube
E. Intraosseous fluid injection

8. A 55-year-old man presents with sudden onset of lower back pain, loss of perineal sensation and urinary incontinence.

What is the SINGLE most *appropriate management*?

A. Admit to hospital
B. Paracetamol and keep active
C. Strict bedrest
D. Skeletal traction
E. Urgent spinal cord decompression

9. A 45-year-old businessman returns from Nigeria with high fever, confusion and rigors.

What is the SINGLE investigation most *likely to give a definitive diagnosis*?

A. Blood cultures
B. Blood film for parasites
C. CT scan of head
D. 12-lead ECG
E. Urine toxicology screen

10. A 30-year-old pregnant woman presents with numbness and tingling in her right hand involving the lateral three fingers.

What is the SINGLE most *appropriate treatment*?

A. Carpal tunnel release surgery
B. Local steroid injection
C. NSAIDs
D. Paracetamol
E. Splinting

11. A 22-year-old man sustains a femoral shaft fracture while rollerblading and is brought to A&E confused and agitated.

What is the SINGLE most *likely diagnosis*?

A. Epidural haematoma
B. Fat embolism
C. Hypovolaemic shock
D. Pericardial effusion
E. Pulmonary embolism

12. A 50-year-old obese man presents with severe central chest pain radiating to his back. He is a heavy smoker and drinker.

    What is the SINGLE most *likely diagnosis*?

    A. Acute myocardial infarction
    B. Acute pericarditis
    C. Dissecting aortic aneurysm
    D. Perforated peptic ulcer
    E. Pulmonary embolism

13. A 30-year-old woman reports palpitations at rest. Resting pulse is 70 and regular. Holter ECG shows irregularities associated with the palpitations.

    What is the SINGLE most *likely diagnosis*?

    A. Atrial fibrillation
    B. Atrial flutter
    C. Heart block
    D. PSVT
    E. Ventricular ectopics

14. A 55-year-old man complains of pleuritic chest pain 5 days after an MI and is found to have persistent ST elevation on ECG. Pain is worse with movement.

    What is the SINGLE most *likely diagnosis*?

    A. Acute pericarditis
    B. Acute pulmonary embolus
    C. Dissecting aortic aneurysm
    D. Dressler syndrome
    E. Ventricular rupture

15. A 35-year-old mother of four reports urinary incontinence. Urometry suggests stress incontinence.

    What is the SINGLE most *appropriate form of treatment*?

    A. Bladder neck surgery
    B. Oxybutynin
    C. Pelvic floor exercises
    D. Pessary
    E. Topical vaginal oestrogens

16. A 7-year-old boy presents with persistent nocturnal enuresis. There is a family history of enuresis. MSU shows no growth.

    What is the SINGLE most *appropriate form of treatment*?

    A. Bladder retraining exercises
    B. Cognitive behavioural therapy
    C. Desmopressin nasal spray
    D. Incontinence pads
    E. Prophylactic dose of trimethoprim

17. A 15-year-old boy presents to A&E with severe asthma. He is using his accessory muscles of respiration and is unable to speak in sentences.

    What is the SINGLE most *appropriate treatment*?

    A. Inhaled short-acting β2 agonist
    B. Inhaled long-acting β2 agonist
    C. IV aminophylline
    D. IV hydrocortisone
    E. Nebulised short-acting β2 agonist

18. A 55-year-old woman post-hysterectomy complains of pleuritic chest pain and coughing up blood.

    What is the SINGLE most *likely diagnosis*?

    A. Acute pericarditis
    B. Atelectasis
    C. Perforated peptic ulcer
    D. Pneumonia
    E. Pulmonary embolism

19. A 40-year-old man presents with BRBPR, constipation and diarrhoea. Sigmoidoscopy reveals an ulcerated stricture in the sigmoid colon.

    What is the SINGLE most *likely diagnosis*?

    A. Angiodysplasia
    B. Crohn's disease
    C. Diverticular disease
    D. Sigmoid colon cancer
    E. Ulcerative colitis

20. A 70-year-old woman presents with dysphagia and regurgitation.

What is the SINGLE investigation most *likely to provide a definitive diagnosis?*

A. Barium swallow
B. Chest x-ray
C. Endoscopy
D. Flexible nasendoscopy
E. Soft-tissue neck x-ray

21. A pedestrian sustains a degloving injury to the lower leg and pelvic fractures. BP is 80/40 and JVP is 2.

What is the SINGLE most *likely diagnosis?*

A. Anaphylactic shock
B. Cardiogenic shock
C. Endocrine failure
D. Gram-negative septicaemia
E. Hypovolaemic shock

22. A 21-year-old university student back from a hiking holiday in Massachusetts presents with bilateral facial nerve palsy and a raised pink annular lesion on her lower leg. She says this was all preceded by flu-like symptoms.

What is the SINGLE most *likely diagnosis?*

A. Erythema multiforme
B. Erythema nodosum
C. Herpes zoster
D. Infected insect bite
E. Lyme disease

23. A 30-year-old man presents with haematuria and BP of 180/100. On exam, you palpate bilateral irregular abdominal masses.

What is the SINGLE investigation most *likely to produce a definitive diagnosis?*

A. CT scan
B. MSU
C. Ultrasound
D. 24-hour urine excretion of 5HIAA
E. 24-hour urine collection for VMA

24. A 50-year-old alcoholic presents with mild jaundice and epistaxis.

What is the SINGLE most *appropriate investigation?*

A. Full blood count
B. Hepatitis virology
C. Liver function tests
D. Platelet count
E. Prothrombin time

25. An insulation company worker presents with cervical lymph nodes and SOB. CXR reveals bilateral pulmonary fibrosis and mild pleural effusion.

What is the SINGLE most *likely diagnosis?*

A. Bronchogenic carcinoma
B. Mesothelioma
C. Sarcoidosis
D. Silicosis
E. Tuberculosis

26. A 15-year-old girl with a neural tube defect is brought in by her mother for advice on urinary incontinence.

What is the SINGLE most *appropriate management?*

A. Desmopressin
B. Incontinence pads
C. Intermittent self-catheterisation
D. Oxybutynin
E. Prophylactic trimethoprim

27. A 38-year-old married working mother of 3 asks for contraception. She states she had a pill-failure in the past and has a history of heavy periods.

What is the SINGLE most *appropriate form of contraception?*

A. Bilateral tubal ligation
B. Condoms
C. Depoprovera injection
D. Mirena coil
E. Norethisterone pop

28. A 56-year-old IDDM male presents with persistently elevated BP of 180/110. Blood tests are unremarkable.

What is the SINGLE most *appropriate medication*?

A. Amlodipine
B. Atenolol
C. Bendrofluazide
D. Frusemide
E. Perindopril

29. A 36-year-old woman is found to have blocked fallopian tubes on laparoscopy and hysterosalpingography. The uterus is normal.

What is the SINGLE most *appropriate next form of treatment*?

A. GnRH agonist
B. Hysteroscopic adhesiolysis
C. Intrauterine insemination
D. In vitro fertilisation
E. Salpingolysis

30. A 30-year-old woman presents with 2 weeks of fever, rigors and productive rusty cough. CXR shows a left lower lobe consolidation.

What is the SINGLE most *likely organism*?

A. *Legionella pneumoniae*
B. *Mycobacterium tuberculosis*
C. *Mycoplasma pneumoniae*
D. *Staphlococcus pneumoniae*
E. *Streptococcus pneumoniae*

31. A 40-year-old man returns from Africa with high swinging pyrexia and diarrhoea. On exam, there is tenderness in the right upper quadrant of the abdomen.

What is the SINGLE most *likely diagnosis*?

A. Acute cholecystitis
B. Acute hepatitis
C. Amoebic liver abscess
D. Falciparum malaria
E. Salmonella poisoning

32. A 58-year-old male heavy smoker states that his right big toe becomes pale and painful when walking.

What is the SINGLE most *likely diagnosis*?

A. Embolism
B. Gout
C. Peripheral atherosclerosis
D. Raynaud's phenomenon
E. Thromboangiitis obliterans

33. A 55-year-old male presents with TIA and is found to have a pulse rate of 100 with irregular rhythm.

What is the SINGLE most *appropriate treatment*?

A. Aspirin
B. DC cardioversion
C. Heparin
D. Streptokinase
E. Warfarin

34. A 33-year-old woman is found to have a solitary 2.5 cm nodule in the left side of the thyroid.

What is the SINGLE most *definitive investigation*?

A. Fine-needle aspirate cytology
B. Serum thyroid function tests
C. Thyroid autoantibodies
D. Thyroid nuclear scanning
E. Ultrasound of thyroid

35. A 50-year-old NIDDM patient brings in a letter from his optician, which states he has extensive proliferative retinopathy.

What is the SINGLE most *definitive treatment*?

A. Add gliclazide to metformin
B. Laser photocoagulation
C. Switch to insulin treatment
D. Topical timolol drops
E. Topical xalatan

36. A 55-year-old naval seaman presents with a rash on his forehead. He states that he has had the rash for years and often forgets to wear his cap while on duty.

What is the SINGLE most *likely diagnosis*?

A. Actinic keratosis
B. Acne vulgaris
C. Keratoacanthoma
D. Lentigo maligna
E. Squamous cell carcinoma

37. A 30-year-old pedestrian involved in a RTA is brought into A&E with loss of consciousness. He regains consciousness and complains of headache, and has neck stiffness on exam. He has a deep laceration to his right temple.

What is the SINGLE most *likely diagnosis*?

A. Basal skull fracture
B. Cerebral haemorrhage
C. Extradural haematoma
D. Subarachnoid haemorrhage
E. Subdural haematoma

38. A 20-year-old cyclist is hit by an oncoming vehicle and now presents with loss of consciousness. On exam, there is blood behind the eardrum and periorbital ecchymoses.

What is the SINGLE most *likely diagnosis*?

A. Basilar skull fracture
B. Extradural haematoma
C. Linear skull fracture
D. Subarachnoid haemorrhage
E. Subdural haematoma

39. A 35-year-old woman complains of severe pain on defecation. She is unable to tolerate digital rectal examination. She has a history of constipation.

What is the SINGLE most *likely diagnosis*?

A. Anal fissure
B. Crohn's disease
C. Haemorrhoids
D. Perianal haematoma
E. Pilonidal cyst

40. A 70-year-old woman being treated for temporal arteritis now presents with fever, severe upper abdominal pain and vomiting.

What is the SINGLE most *likely diagnosis?*

A. Acute cholecystitis
B. Acute pancreatitis
C. Gallstone peritonitis
D. Perforated peptic ulcer
E. Ruptured aortic aneurysm

41. A 50-year-old Iranian farmer presents with fever, rigors and hepatosplenomegaly.

What is the SINGLE most *likely diagnosis?*

A. Brucellosis
B. Hepatitis
C. Malaria
D. Tuberculosis
E. Typhoid fever

42. A 55-year-old man presents with prostatic symptoms. On digital rectal exam, you palpate a firm nodule on the prostate.

What is the next SINGLE most *appropriate investigation?*

A. Acid phosphatase
B. IVU
C. Scintiscan
D. Serum PSA levels
E. Transrectal ultrasound

43. A 45-year-old man with a history of heart failure now presents with moderate to severe depression.

What is the SINGLE most *appropriate treatment?*

A. Amitriptyline
B. Cognitive behavioural therapy
C. Exercise three times weekly
D. Fluoxetine
E. Venlafaxine

44. A 15-year-old girl is brought in by her family as they are concerned she is anorexic and depressed. BMI is 15. She has no suicidal ideation.

What is the SINGLE most *appropriate treatment*?

A. Commence fluoxetine
B. Offer cognitive behavioural therapy
C. Refer to rapid access mental health team
D. Section and admit to hospital
E. Suggest family counselling

45. A 40-year-old triathlon athlete complains of pain in his side. He cannot keep still.

What is the SINGLE investigation most *likely to provide a definitive diagnosis*?

A. AXR
B. CXR
C. MSU
D. Ultrasound
E. Urinalysis

46. A 30-year-old man with ankylosing spondylitis now presents with eye pain and redness.

What is the SINGLE most *likely diagnosis*?

A. Acute angle closure glaucoma
B. Acute conjunctivitis
C. Herpetic ulcer
D. Iritis
E. Scleritis

47. A 10-year-old boy has SOB and wheezing when playing football.

What is the SINGLE most *appropriate treatment*?

A. Inhaled steroids
B. Nebulised salbutamol
C. Sodium cromoglycate
D. Trial of leukotriene receptor antagonist
E. Trial of short-acting β2 agonist

48. A 60-year-old man presents with severe SOB with basal crepitation on auscultation. BP is 160/110 with a pulse of 100. CXR confirms suspicions.

What is the SINGLE most *appropriate treatment*?

A. Amlodipine
B. Bendrofluazide
C. Frusemide
D. Nifedipine
E. Spironolactone

49. A 25-year-old man complains of bouts of alternating intermittent diarrhoea and constipation for the past month. He describes a sensation of incomplete evacuation and bloating. Symptoms are relieved by defecation. Sigmoidoscopy is normal.

What is the SINGLE most *likely diagnosis*?

A. Diverticulosis
B. Gastroenteritis
C. Irritable bowel syndrome
D. Pseudomembranous colitis
E. Ulcerative colitis

50. A 50-year-old man post-op cholecystectomy presents with fever, jaundice and dark urine.

What is the SINGLE most *definitive management*?

A. Abdominal ultrasound
B. CT scan
C. ERCP
D. Laparotomy
E. Percutaneous transhepatic cholangiography

51. A 26-year-old man with NIDDM and a history of haemochromatosis now presents with jaundice.

What is the SINGLE most *definitive investigation*?

A. Abdominal ultrasound
B. ERCP
C. Liver biopsy
D. Serum ferritin levels
E. Viral hepatitis serology

52. A 9-month-old baby is brought in to A&E, as the baby is inconsolable. The mother notes that the baby has a distended abdomen and reports that the baby is vomiting and cannot keep food down. AXR shows a transverse line just below the umbilicus.

What is the SINGLE most *likely diagnosis*?

A. Hirschsprung's disease
B. Intussusception
C. Meckel's diverticulum
D. Pyloric stenosis
E. Toxic megacolon

53. A 55-year-old man with new-onset dyspepsia reports no relief with antacids.

What is the SINGLE most *appropriate management*?

A. Arrange barium meal
B. Refer urgently for endoscopy
C. Test for *Helicobacter pylori*
D. Trial of lansoprazole
E. 24-hour ambulatory oesophageal pH monitoring

54. A 69-year-old man with a history of intermittent claudication now reports severe back pain. On exam, BP is 90/50.

What is the SINGLE most *definitive investigation*?

A. Abdominal ultrasound
B. CXR
C. 12-lead ECG
D. Spiral CT scan
E. MRI spine

55. A 50-year-old woman post oesophagectomy for oesophageal carcinoma presents with a BP of 80/50 in the recovery room. She is on a morphine drip for pain. Hb is 10 gm/dl. She suddenly loses consciousness.

What is the SINGLE most *likely diagnosis*?

A. Acute peritonitis
B. Acute pulmonary embolism
C. DIC
D. Loss of splenic artery ligature
E. Septicaemia

56. A 30-year-old man presents with bloody diarrhoea and mucus stools. Histology shows crypt abscesses and granular inflammatory mucosa.

What is the SINGLE most *likely diagnosis*?

A. Angiodysplasia
B. Crohn's disease
C. Diverticular disease
D. Irritable bowel syndrome
E. Ulcerative colitis

57. A 50-year-old man is brought into A&E after overdosing on his pills. No label is found on the bottle. The patient is noted to be in heart block, and has a palpable bladder and dilated pupils.

What is the SINGLE most *likely culprit*?

A. Coproxamol
B. Fluoxetine
C. Quinine
D. Tricyclic antidepressant
E. Venlafaxine

58. An 80-year-old woman notes that she had trouble putting up her curtains yesterday evening. She states she loses her balance and falls.

What is the SINGLE most *definitive investigation*?

A. Cervical x-ray
B. Hallpike manoeuvre
C. Hearing test
D. Measurement of intraocular pressures
E. Visual acuity

59. A 1-year-old develops swollen lips after eating peanuts.

What is the SINGLE most *appropriate management*?

A. Administer IM adrenaline
B. Administer IV hydrocortisone
C. Administer IV chlorphenamine
D. Admit to hospital urgently
E. Prescribe oral antihistamine

60. A 30-year-old woman develops bilateral conductive hearing loss after giving birth. On examination the tympanic membranes appear normal.

What is the SINGLE most *likely diagnosis*?

A. Acoustic neuroma
B. Acute otitis media
C. Gentamicin toxicity
D. Ménière's disease
E. Otosclerosis

61. An 8-year-old boy is suspected to be allergic to strawberries.

What is the SINGLE most *appropriate investigation*?

A. Double-blind, placebo-controlled food provocation challenge
B. Skin prick test
C. Radio-allergo-sorbant test
D. Tissue transglutaminase antibody
E. Total IgE blood test

62. A 22-year-old man reports that he was bitten by a stray dog.

What is the SINGLE most *appropriate management*?

A. Clean wound and give co-amoxyclavulanic acid
B. Clean wound, infiltrate wound with human rabies immunoglobulin half into the wound and half IM and administer rabies vaccine IM on days 0, 3, 7, 14, 30 and 90
C. Clean wound and notify NSPCA to catch dog, quarantine and observe whether dog develops rabies
D. Clean wound and reassure
E. Clean wound and administer rabies vaccine IM on days 0, 3, 7, 14, 30 and 90

63. A 60-year-old married woman is brought in by her husband as he reports that she is behaving oddly. She has suddenly been making inappropriate sexual remarks in public. She has always been a shy person and now is extremely extrovert.

What is the SINGLE most *likely diagnosis*?

A. Alzheimer's disease
B. Delirium
C. Frontal lobe lesion
D. Subdural haematoma
E. Tourette's syndrome

64. A 10-year-old boy is brought into Casualty in the British Isles by his parents following a weaver fish sting on the local beach.

What is the SINGLE most *appropriate treatment*?

A. Administer paracetamol suspension
B. Administer ibuprofen suspension
C. Administer antihistamines
D. Clean wound and administer paracetamol
E. Immerse in hot water for 15 minutes

65. A 30-year-old female complains of persistent fever and diarrhoea. On examination she is noted to have a fistulo in ano and perianal skin tags.

What is the SINGLE most *likely diagnosis*?

A. Crohn's disease
B. Gastroenteritis
C. Haemorrhoids
D. Irritable bowel syndrome
E. Ulcerative colitis

66. A 50-year-old man complains of pain on defecation. On examination there is a tender reddish blue swelling near the anal verge.

What is the SINGLE most *likely diagnosis*?

A. Fistulo-in-ano
B. Haemorrhoids
C. Perianal abscess
D. Perianal haematoma
E. Pilonidal cyst

67. An 8-year-old boy is wheelchair bound with a neural tube defect. He is found to be persistently incontinent of urine. MSU shows no growth.

What is the SINGLE most *appropriate management*?

A. Desmopressin nasal spray
B. Foley catheter attached to leg bag
C. Incontinence pants
D. Intermittent self-catheterisation
E. Long-term prophylactic trimethoprim

68. A 25-year-old bicyclist was struck by a car and presents with perineal bruising. He has been unable to void for the past 2 hours. On rectal exam, his prostate is noted to be high-riding.

What is the SINGLE most *appropriate management*?

A. Arrange retrograde urethrogram
B. Arrange IVU
C. Insert foley catheter
D. Insert suprapubic catheter
E. Obtain pelvic x-ray

69. A 30-year-old banker complains of headaches and blurry vision. He sits in front of his VDU screen for 8 hours a day checking the stock market.

What is the SINGLE most *appropriate investigation*?

A. ESR
B. Intraocular pressure
C. Split lamp test
D. Refer to optician for visual acuity testing
E. Visual field test

70. A 70-year-old woman reports tunnel vision and seeing haloes around lights with vision worse in the evening.

What is the SINGLE most *appropriate investigation*?

A. ESR
B. Intraocular pressure
C. Split lamp test
D. Refer to optician for visual acuity testing
E. Visual field test

71. A 77-year-old man reports difficulty reading the newspaper with missing words, seeing straight lines as wavy and an empty spot in the centre of his vision.

What is the SINGLE most *likely diagnosis*?

A. Acute glaucoma
B. Age-related macular degeneration
C. Cataract
D. Central retinal vein thrombosis
E. Optic neuritis

72. A 10-year-old child presents with 15% body surface area burns.

    What is the SINGLE most *appropriate management*?

    A. Administer IVFs, clean, dress wounds in A&E and discharge
    B. Admit, notify social services, puncture blisters and perform escharo-tomy as needed
    C. Irrigate with cold water, dress wounds and discharge with silver sul-fadiazine and dressings
    D. Clean, use dry occlusive dressings and discharge on broad-spectrum antibiotics
    E. Refer to specialist burns unit

73. A 55-year-old woman presents with a plaque-like lesion on her lower calf and a painless ulcer on the sole of her foot.

    What is the SINGLE most *useful investigation*?

    A. ESR
    B. Fasting blood glucose
    C. Lyme disease serology
    D. Peripheral arteriogram
    E. Skin biopsy

74. A 50-year-old woman complains of tinnitus, vertigo and deafness. It is so disabling that she is house-bound. Deafness improves gradually.

    What is the SINGLE most *likely diagnosis*?

    A. Acoustic neuroma
    B. Ménière's disease
    C. Otosclerosis
    D. Presbyacusis
    E. Viral labyrinthitis

75. An 80-year-old female resident of a nursing home is seen in Casualty for generalised bruising. A month prior she was admitted for a femoral neck fracture sustained falling out of bed. A year ago she sustained a Colles fracture after tripping over her feet.

    What is the SINGLE most *likely diagnosis*?

    A. Balance disorder
    B. Non-accidental injury
    C. Osteoporosis
    D. Postural hypotension
    E. Vitamin K deficiency

76. A 45-year-old alcoholic male would like medication to help him abstain from drinking. He attends AA and has been sober for 1 week.

What is the SINGLE most *useful treatment*?

A. Acamprosate
B. Chlormethiazole
C. Diazepam
D. Disulfiram
E. Lorazepam

77. A 40-year-old woman suffering from asthma is also noted to be hyperthyroid.

What is the SINGLE most *appropriate management*?

A. Commence carbimazole
B. Commence Lugol's iodine
C. Commence propranolol
D. Commence thyroxine
E. Refer for thyroidectomy

78. A 75-year-old female resident of a nursing home presents with intractable itching. On exam, there are burrows between her fingers.

What is the SINGLE most *appropriate management*?

A. Treat with 25% benzyl benzoate
B. Treat with 1% carbaryl
C. Treat with 0.5% malathion lotion
D. Treat with 5% permethrin
E. Treat with 0.5% phenothrin

79. A 4-day-old breast-fed baby presents with jaundice. The mother is concerned, as her baby has also lost 250 g in weight. Stools are not pale.

What is the SINGLE most *likely diagnosis*?

A. Biliary atresia
B. Breast-feeding jaundice
C. Breast milk jaundice
D. Galactosaemia
E. Rh incompatibility

80. A 17-day-old breast-fed baby presents with jaundice. The mother is concerned, as the stools are clay-coloured.

What is the SINGLE most *likely diagnosis*?

A. Biliary atresia
B. Breast-feeding jaundice
C. Breast milk jaundice
D. Galactosaemia
E. Rh incompatibility

81. A 1-week-old boy is brought to Casualty by his Korean father, as he is concerned about a nontender bluish patch on the baby's right buttock cheek. He is worried, as his wife is suffering from postnatal depression.

What is the SINGLE most *likely diagnosis*?

A. Bleeding disorder
B. Child neglect
C. Mongolian spot
D. Naevus
E. Non-accidental injury

82. A 5-year-old boy is noted to have a clumsy gait and mild scoliosis. When he gets up off the floor, he uses his hands to climb up his legs.

What is the SINGLE most *likely diagnosis*?

A. Duchenne's muscular dystrophy
B. Guillain–Barré syndrome
C. Hunter's syndrome
D. Motor neurone disease
E. Polio

83. A 5-year-old girl presents after a fall on her right arm off a swing. On examination there is no swelling or deformity, but the forearm is extremely tender.

What is the SINGLE most *likely diagnosis*?

A. Greenstick fracture
B. Non-accidental injury
C. Pulled elbow (subluxation of the radial head)
D. Smith's fracture
E. Spiral fracture

84. A 6-year-old girl is brought into Casualty by her nanny, complaining of arm pain and inability to use her arm. The nanny explains that she was twirling the child around like an aeroplane.

What is the SINGLE most *likely diagnosis*?

A. Fracture of radius/ulna
B. Greenstick fracture
C. Non-accidental injury
D. Pulled elbow (subluxation of the radial head)
E. Spiral fracture

85. A 6-week-old baby is brought in by her mother, who is concerned as the baby is always hungry and cannot keep milk down. Mother denies that the baby has been vomiting bile. On examination, a small mass is palpated in the upper abdomen.

What is the SINGLE most *likely diagnosis*?

A. Coeliac disease
B. Gastroenteritis
C. GERD
D. Intussusception
E. Pyloric stenosis

86. A 14-year-old boy complains of sudden pain in his groin after cycling 10 miles.

What is the SINGLE most *likely diagnosis*?

A. Femoral hernia
B. Pulled muscle
C. Testicular torsion
D. Urethral trauma
E. Varicocoele

87. A 50-year-old burns victim needs to be commenced on IV fluids.

What is the SINGLE most *appropriate type of fluid*?

A. Colloid solution
B. Crystalloid (Ringer's lactate)
C. Dextrose water
D. Normal saline
E. Plasmalyte

88. A 16-year-old girl who had recently had a sore throat now complains of severe left-sided upper abdominal pain. On examination, there is pallor. BP 60/40 P130. Abdomen is tense and rigid, with no bowel sounds.

What is the SINGLE most *likely diagnosis*?

A. Acute pyelonephritis
B. Fitz-Hugh–Curtis syndrome
C. Perforated peptic ulcer
D. Peritonitis
E. Ruptured spleen

89. A 4-year-old girl presents with nasal speech and snoring. The mother is concerned as the child is somnolent during the day and the teachers find her inattentive.

What is the SINGLE most *appropriate management*?

A. Prescribe ephedrine nasal drops
B. Reassure mother that child will outgrow this
C. Refer for pure tone audiogram
D. Refer for assessment for tonsillectomy and adenoidectomy
E. Refer to child psychiatry

90. A 5-year-old child is brought in by the mother, as she is concerned that the child is falling behind at school. She thinks the child's hearing may be affected. The child has no earache. On examination, tympanic membranes are dull.

What is the SINGLE most *likely diagnosis*?

A. ADHD
B. Chronic otitis media
C. Developmental delay
D. Eustachian tube dysfunction
E. Otitis externa

91. A 29-year-old woman, with a family history of breast cancer in her mother at age 35, would like to be screened for breast carcinoma.

What is the SINGLE most *appropriate management*?

A. Offer mammogram
B. Offer ultrasound
C. Reassurance as no breast symptoms at present
D. Refer to family history breast clinic
E. Urgent referral to one-stop breast clinic

92. A 60-year-old man complains of blurred speech and weakness, and tingling of his left arm. The episode lasted 3 hours.

What is the SINGLE investigation *likely to give a definitive diagnosis*?

A. CT scan of head
B. Doppler ultrasound of carotids
C. EEG
D. MRI scan
E. 12-lead ECG

93. A 40-year-old woman complains of pain on sideways movement of her eyes and decreased colour vision.

What is the SINGLE most *likely diagnosis*?

A. Central retinal artery occlusion
B. Central retinal vein occlusion
C. Giant cell arteritis
D. Glaucoma
E. Optic neuritis

94. A 70-year-old man on the Geriatric ward develops confusion. On exam, the bladder is palpable at the umbilicus.

What is the SINGLE most *likely explanation*?

A. Acute renal failure
B. Alzheimer's disease
C. Delirium secondary to UTI
D. Senile dementia
E. Urinary retention secondary to prostatic hypertrophy

95. A 50-year-old woman reports an episode of sudden loss of consciousness. She only recalls her heart thumping prior to the event and her face looking flushed upon recovery.

What is the SINGLE most *likely diagnosis*?

A. Carotid sinus syndrome
B. Epilepsy
C. Stokes-Adams attack
D. Stroke
E. TIA

96. A 75-year-old woman becomes increasingly forgetful. She suffers from the most common form of dementia, a dementia characterised by neurofibrillary tangles and senile plaques.

    What is the SINGLE most *likely form of dementia*?

    A. Alzheimer's disease
    B. Multi-infarct dementia
    C. Parkinson's disease
    D. Pseudodementia
    E. Senile dementia

97. A 77-year-old man notices that he has trouble finding the right word and composing sentences. He also gets recurrent partial paralysis on the right side of his body.

    What is the SINGLE most *likely diagnosis*?

    A. Alzheimer's disease
    B. Frontal dementia
    C. Lewy body dementia
    D. Parkinson's disease
    E. Vascular dementia

98. A 65-year-old woman reports headache and scalp tenderness when she combs her hair.

    What is the SINGLE most *appropriate initial investigation*?

    A. CT scan head
    B. ESR
    C. Platelets
    D. Slit lamp exam
    E. Temporal artery biopsy

99. A 65-year-old woman with a history of rheumatoid arthritis now presents with epistaxis. Blood tests reveal a pancytopaenia. On exam, there is no blood PR.

    What is the SINGLE most *likely diagnosis*?

    A. Anaemia of chronic disease
    B. Aplastic anaemia
    C. ITP
    D. Reaction to NSAIDs
    E. Reaction to methotrexate

100. A 50-year-old woman post thyroidectomy complains of tingling around her lips.

What is the SINGLE most *useful investigation*?

A. CT scan of head
B. Serum calcium levels
C. Serum thyroid function tests
D. Serum urea and electrolytes
E. Ultrasound of neck

101. A 12-year-old boy is brought in by his mother for recurrent epistaxis. On exam, there is crusting in the nasal vestibule.

What is the SINGLE most *appropriate treatment*?

A. Flucloxacillin
B. Fusidic ointment
C. Neomycin cream
D. Silver nitrate cauterisation
E. Topical beconase steroid spray

102. A 30-year-old woman exhibits pressured speech and flight of ideas, changing subjects frequently in conversation.

What is the SINGLE most *likely diagnosis*?

A. Dementia
B. Mania
C. Obsessive compulsive disorder
D. Paranoia
E. Schizophrenia

103. A 55-year-old man with asthma was recently started on an antihypertensive drug, which he now thinks is responsible for his impotence.

What is the SINGLE most *likely culprit*?

A. Amlodipine
B. Atenolol
C. Bendrofluazide
D. Frusemide
E. Perindopril

104. A 56-year-old man binges on food and alcohol and suddenly develops massive haematemesis.

What is the SINGLE most *likely diagnosis*?

A. Alcoholic cirrhosis
B. Gastric erosion
C. Mallory-Weiss tear
D. Perforated peptic ulcer
E. Ruptured aortic aneurysm

105. A 60-year-old man requires add-on therapy to manage his hypertension. BP is persistently elevated at 175/110 on maximum doses of atenolol. He has a history of gout.

What is the SINGLE most *appropriate drug treatment*?

A. Amlodipine
B. Bendrofluazide
C. Frusemide
D. Losartan
E. Perindopril

106. A 55-year-old Middle Eastern man returns from the Hajj pilgrimage complaining of fever, rigor, myalgia, weight loss, diarrhoea and pain in his joints. On examination, both the liver and spleen are palpable. Blood tests show a pancytopaenia.

What is the SINGLE most *likely diagnosis*?

A. Brucellosis
B. Cholera
C. Malaria
D. Shigella
E. Typhoid fever

107. A 20-year-old American exchange student from Idaho presents with high fever, rigors, severe frontal headache, photophobia and reports that 4 days later a rash appeared on his palms and soles. On examination, the spleen is palpable.

What is the SINGLE most *likely diagnosis*?

A. Hand foot and mouth disease
B. Lyme disease
C. Rocky Mountain spotted fever
D. Syphilis
E. Tuberculosis

108. A 6-year-old girl is brought in by her grandmother as she noted blood in the girl's knickers. The grandmother explains that the girl's mother gives a story of falling off a bicycle.

What is the SINGLE most *likely diagnosis?*

A. Premature puberty
B. Renal colic
C. Sexual abuse
D. Urethral trauma
E. UTI

109. An 80-year-old woman is noted to have unilateral right-sided tonsillar hypertrophy.

What is the SINGLE most *likely diagnosis?*

A. Lymphoma
B. Peritonsillar cellulitis
C. Quinsy
D. Tonsil carcinoma
E. Viral tonsillitis

110. A 65-year-old woman requests medication for the prevention of osteoporosis. She is on long-term prednisolone for PMR.

What is the SINGLE most *appropriate medication?*

A. Bisphosphonates
B. Calcitonin
C. Disodium etidronate
D. HRT
E. Raloxifene

111. A 35-year-old man with schizophrenia develops galactor-rhoea.

What is the SINGLE most *appropriate investigation?*

A. CT scan of head
B. Drug levels of antipsychotic
C. Ductogram
D. Serum prolactin
E. Urea and electrolytes

112. A 60-year-old obese female is admitted for elective total hip replacement.

    What is the SINGLE most *important pre-operative treatment*?

    A. Chest PT
    B. IV fluids
    C. Rectal suppository
    D. SC heparin
    E. Ted stockings

113. A 70-year-old man presents with both back pain and acute renal failure.

    What is the SINGLE most *likely diagnosis*?

    A. IgA nephropathy
    B. Metastatic prostate carcinoma
    C. Multiple myeloma
    D. Poststreptococcal glomerulonephritis
    E. Sarcoidosis

114. A 45-year-old obese woman reports right shoulder pain 30 minutes after eating meals.

    What is the SINGLE investigation most *likely to give a definitive diagnosis*?

    A. Abdominal x-ray
    B. Abdominal ultrasound
    C. CT scan of abdomen
    D. Upper GI endoscopy
    E. Upright chest x-ray

115. A 60-year-old alcoholic male now presents with severe abdominal pain and vomiting. On examination, T = 40°C, and the abdomen is tense, distended and rigid, with no bowel sounds.

    What is the SINGLE investigation most *likely to give a definitive diagnosis*?

    A. Abdominal x-ray
    B. Abdominal ultrasound
    C. CT scan abdomen
    D. Upper GI endoscopy
    E. Upright chest x-ray

116. An 80-year-old male resident of a nursing home presents with urinary retention. On examination, the bladder is distended and the sigmoid colon is palpable.

What is the SINGLE most *likely diagnosis*?

A. Benign prostatic hypertrophy
B. Diverticulosis
C. Faecal impaction
D. Sigmoid colon carcinoma
E. UTI

117. A 55-year-old alcoholic man complains of severe upper abdominal pain radiating to the back, loose, pale stools and weight loss. AXR shows calcifications.

What is the SINGLE most *likely diagnosis*?

A. Acute pancreatitis
B. Chronic pancreatitis
C. GERD
D. Oesophagitis
E. Pancreatitic carcinoma

118. A 50-year-old man reports that he can only swallow liquids and solids slowly. CXR reveals an air–fluid level behind the heart.

What is the SINGLE most *likely diagnosis*?

A. Achalasia
B. Barrett's oesophagus
C. Bulbar palsy
D. GERD
E. Globus pharyngeus

119. A 50-year-old man reports that he has difficulty swallowing and when he does, he coughs.

What is the SINGLE most *likely diagnosis*?

A. Achalasia
B. Barrett's oesophagus
C. Bulbar palsy
D. GERD
E. Globus pharyngeus

120. A 30-year-old heroin addict presents with purple papules in his mouth and on his lower leg.

What is the SINGLE most *likely diagnosis?*

A. Henoch-Schönlein purpura
B. Kaposi's sarcoma
C. Lichen planus
D. Malignant melanoma
E. TTP

121. A 50-year-old man presents with fever, night sweats, malaise, weight loss and itching. On examination, he also has bruises, gout and a palpable liver and spleen. FBC shows raised WCC, platelets and red cell mass.

What is the SINGLE most *likely explanation?*

A. Bone marrow infiltration
B. Decreased red blood cell survival
C. Erythropoietin deficiency
D. Haemolysis
E. Myeloproliferative disorder

122. A 30-year-old male flight attendant presents with a painless left red eye. He states that he has had this red eye for 6 weeks. On examination, there is redness over the temporal region of the left conjunctiva. Visual acuity is normal.

What is the SINGLE most *likely diagnosis?*

A. Episcleritis
B. Hyphaema
C. Kaposi's sarcoma
D. Subconjunctival haemorrhage
E. Vitreous haemorrhage

123. A 25-year-old fire-fighter presents to A&E with a painful throat and coughing up black sputum. He states that he was in a confined space in a burning building for 20 minutes. On examination, the eyebrows and nose hairs in the vestibule are singed. He becomes disoriented.

What is the SINGLE most *appropriate management?*

A. Anaesthetise and endotracheal intubation
B. Analgesia
C. Arterial blood gas with carboxyhaemoglobin levels
D. High flow oxygen via a non-rebreathing mask
E. Surgical tracheostomy

124. A 20-year-old woman presents with intermenstrual bleeding. She was started on Microgynon 4 months ago. She has a new partner.

What is the SINGLE most *relevant investigation*?

A. Endocervical and high vaginal swabs
B. Endometrial sampling
C. Pap smear
D. Transvaginal ultrasound
E. Urine for chlamydia

125. A 40-year-old female complains of constipation, malaise, polydipsia, polyuria and weight loss. FBG is 5 mmol/l.

What is the SINGLE most *likely diagnosis*?

A. Chronic renal failure
B. Colon carcinoma
C. Diabetes mellitus
D. Hypercalcaemia
E. Irritable bowel syndrome

126. A 28-year-old man presents with a 2-week history of a painful swollen right knee. On examination, he is found to have iritis and non-specific urethritis. A month prior he had a severe bout of diarrhoea.

What is the SINGLE most *appropriate treatment*?

A. Allopurinol
B. Ciprofloxacin
C. Colchicine
D. Naproxen
E. Paracetamol

127. A 22-year-old woman presents with 2 months of recurrent bouts of fever and diarrhoea. She reports that she sees blood and mucus in her stool. She has been losing weight.

What is the SINGLE investigation most *likely to lead to a definitive diagnosis*?

A. ESR
B. Proctoscopy
C. Sigmoidoscopy
D. Stool for culture and microscopy for ova and parasites
E. Stool for occult blood

128. A 7-year-old girl falls onto an outstretched hand. On examination, the radial pulse is absent.

What is the SINGLE most *likely diagnosis*?

A. Colles fracture
B. Fracture of clavicle
C. Greenstick fracture
D. Scaphoid fracture
E. Supracondylar fracture of humerus

129. An 18-month-old baby is brought in with dehydration from diarrhoea and vomiting for the past 72 hours.

What is the SINGLE most *useful treatment*?

A. D5W
B. 0.9% saline
C. Oral rehydration solution (60 mmol)
D. Oral rehydration solution (90 mmol)
E. Water by mouth

130. A 6-year-old girl is brought in by her mother for recurrent vomiting and dehydration. Mother reports that the child vomits 5× an hour for hours at a time for the past 4 days. She is concerned. There is a family history of migraines. The parents recently divorced. On examination, the abdomen is nad.

What is the SINGLE most *likely diagnosis*?

A. Attention-seeking behaviour
B. Bulimia
C. Cyclical vomiting syndrome
D. UTI
E. Viral gastritis

131. A 9-month-old baby is brought into A&E. The mother is concerned as her baby is inconsolable. Her baby has been vomiting and cannot keep food down. On examination, the abdomen is distended and a sausage-shaped mass is palpable.

What is the SINGLE investigation most *likely to give a definitive diagnosis*?

A. Abdominal ultrasound
B. Abdominal x-ray
C. Barium enema
D. CT scan of abdomen
E. Proctoscopy

132. A 50-year-old man has recently had an uncomplicated myocardial infarction. He would like to know how many days after an MI is he allowed to travel by air.

What is the SINGLE *best answer*?

A. 72 hours
B. 7 days
C. 10 days
D. 14 days
E. 28 days

133. The mother of a 2-year-old boy is worried that he is not speaking in sentences yet.

What is the SINGLE most *appropriate management*?

A. Normal development, so reassure
B. Refer for audiometry
C. Refer to child psychiatry
D. Refer to community paediatrician for milestone assessment
E. Refer for speech therapy

134. A 20-year-old man presents with fever and testicular pain. On examination, a tender red swelling is palpable that is separate from the testes with scrotal oedema.

What is the SINGLE most *useful investigation*?

A. Early morning cultures for Tb
B. MSU for culture and sensitivities
C. Ultrasound
D. Urethral swab
E. Urethrography

135. A 45-year-old man complains of a dragging sensation in his groin. On examination, when standing, the scrotum hangs lower on the affected side and the affected testes is smaller. The pain disappears on lying down.

What is the SINGLE most *likely diagnosis*?

A. Acute epididymo-orchitis
B. Hydrocoele
C. Inguinal hernia
D. Testicular torsion
E. Varicocoele

136. A 13-year-old female pedestrian is involved in a hit and run. She presents with comminuted tib/fib fractures of her lower right leg. On examination, the dorsalis pedis and posterior tibial pulses are absent on the right and there is paralysis of dorsiflexion with foot drop.

What is the SINGLE next most *important management*?

A. Amputation
B. Arteriography and pressure measurements
C. Continuous IV heparin infusion
D. Femoral embolectomy
E. Prophylactic fasciotomy

137. A 60-year-old man post total hip replacement is noted to have a high fever, BP of 100/60 and warm peripheries.

What is the SINGLE most *appropriate investigation*?

A. Arterial blood gas
B. Blood cultures
C. CXR
D. Full blood count
E. V/Q scan

138. A 65-year-old man presents with dribbling, nocturia, and hesitancy. PSA is elevated.

What is the SINGLE most *appropriate investigation*?

A. CT scan
B. Radionuclide bone scan
C. Transrectal ultrasound
D. TRUS-guided biopsy
E. TURP

139. A 30-year-old man postop. day 2 of appendicectomy presents with swinging pyrexia and abdominal pain. On examination, there is tenderness and swelling around the surgical site.

What is the SINGLE most *appropriate investigation*?

A. Abdominal ultrasound
B. AXR
C. Blood cultures
D. CXR
E. Needle aspiration

140. A 70-year-old male presents with severe BRBPR and abdominal pain. BP is 100/60 P 120.

What is the SINGLE investigation most *likely to give a definitive diagnosis*?

A. Angiography
B. Barium enema
C. CT scan of abdomen
D. Colonoscopy
E. Ultrasound of abdomen

141. A 12-year-old girl presents with recurrent epistaxis and crusting in her nose.

What is the SINGLE most *likely diagnosis*?

A. Allergic rhinitis
B. Nasal vestibulitis
C. Perennial rhinitis
D. Rhinosinusitis
E. Wegener's granulomatosis

142. A 50-year-old woman presents with suspected carpal tunnel syndrome.

What is the SINGLE most *common finding on examination*?

A. Atrophy of thenar eminence
B. Loss of sensation over the thenar eminence
C. Weakness of abductor pollicis brevis
D. Weakness of the flexor pollicis brevis
E. Weakness of opponens pollicis

143. A 50-year-old woman is found to have microcalcifications on her mammogram.

What is the SINGLE most *appropriate investigation*?

A. Cone biopsy
B. Excisional biopsy
C. Fine-needle aspirate cytology
D. Stereotactic biopsy
E. Ultrasound

144. A 70-year-old woman reports pain in both buttocks and thigh after walking 100 m. The pain is relieved by rest and sitting down. On examination SLR is negative but pain is elicited on back extension.

What is the SINGLE most *likely diagnosis*?

A. Central disc prolapse
B. L4–L5 disc prolapse
C. Mechanical back pain
D. Spinal stenosis
E. Vertebral fracture

145. A 40-year-old man presents with headache and loss of temporal vision in both eyes. He states that his wedding band does not fit anymore; his fingers are too big.

What is the SINGLE most *useful investigation*?

A. Carotid doppler
B. CT scan of head
C. MRI scan pituitary
D. MRI scan temporal lobe
E. Slit lamp exam of fundi with IOPs

146. A 1-year-old girl has a grand mal seizure with tongue biting and incontinence.

What is the SINGLE *gold standard investigation of choice*?

A. Blood tests
B. EEG
C. MRI scan
D. PET
E. SPECT

147. A 12-year-old girl presents with a non-blanching rash. She is commenced on IV benzylpenicillin. However she remains febrile and is now becoming drowsy.

What is the SINGLE most *appropriate management*?

A. Blood culture
B. Change IV antibiotic to chloramphenicol
C. CT scan of head
D. IV fluids
E. Lumbar puncture

148. A 70-year-old man presents with lower back pain following a fall. The pain is worse at night and is not relieved by simple analgesia. He is in acute urinary retention and reports months of dribbling, hesitancy and nocturia.

What is the SINGLE most *likely diagnosis*?

A. Central disc prolapse
B. Mechanical back pain
C. Metastatic prostate carcinoma
D. Multiple myeloma
E. Sciatica

149. A 50-year-old woman presents with greasy, sticky, smelly stools. Blood tests reveal a macrocytic anaemia.

What is the SINGLE most *likely diagnosis*?

A. Coeliac disease
B. Cirrhosis
C. Irritable bowel syndrome
D. Pernicious anamia
E. Sideroblastic anaemia

150. A 15-year-old girl has marked dehydration from a severe bout of glandular fever. You are unable to gain peripheral IV access for both fluids and antibiotics.

What is the SINGLE most *appropriate management*?

A. Central line insertion
B. Intraosseous injection
C. NG tube insertion
D. Saphenous vein cutdown
E. Subcutaneous fluids

151. A 60-year-old woman complains of headache, right eye pain and blurry vision when closing her curtains that evening. On examination, the pupil is dilated and sluggish.

What is the SINGLE investigation most *likely to yield a definitive diagnosis*?

A. Auscultation for carotid bruits
B. ESR
C. Fluorescein stain
D. Intraocular pressure
E. MRI scan

152. A 20-year-old woman presents with recurrent epistaxis. On examination, there are visible vessels in Little's area.

    What is the SINGLE most *appropriate management*?

    A. Anterior nasal pack with 4 cm merocel
    B. Anterior nasal pack with 8 cm merocel
    C. Brighton balloon tamponade
    D. Naseptin cream
    E. Silver nitrate cautery

153. A 55-year-old man reports the worst headache of his life centred around his right eye. He denies head trauma. On examination, there is neck stiffness. He starts vomiting, feeling faint and eventually becomes drowsy while in Casualty.

    What is the SINGLE most *likely diagnosis*?
    A. Extradural haematoma
    B. Migraine
    C. Periorbital abscess
    D. Subarachnoid haemorrhage
    E. Subdural haematoma

154. A 30-year-old coal miner presents with singed nose hairs and eyebrows.

    What is the SINGLE most *likely diagnosis*?

    A. Arsenic poisoning
    B. Carbon monoxide poisoning
    C. Severe sunburn
    D. Silicosis
    E. Solar keratosis

155. A 55-year-old man complains of retrosternal burning pain radiating to the neck, made worse by hot and cold foods. He also complains of dysphagia and regurgitation.

    What is the SINGLE most *likely diagnosis*?

    A. Achalasia
    B. Barrett's ulcer
    C. GERD
    D. Oesophageal carcinoma
    E. Pharyngeal pouch

156. A 45-year-old man complains of epigastric pain radiating to the back, which is worse at night and relieved with food.

What is the SINGLE most *likely diagnosis*?

A. Barrett's ulcer
B. Duodenal ulcer
C. Gastric ulcer
D. GERD
E. Pancreatitis

157. A 40-year-old male presents with fever, malaise and skin nodules. On examination, BP is 180/100. Presence of splinter haemorrhages is noted and red cells in his urine.

What is the SINGLE most *likely diagnosis*?

A. Adult polycystic kidneys
B. Berger's disease (IgA nephropathy)
C. Polyarteritis nodosa
D. Rheumatoid arthritis
E. Sarcoidosis

158. A NIDDM with renal disease is noted to have a persistently elevated BP of 180/110.

What is the SINGLE most *appropriate medication*?

A. ACE inhibitor
B. Angiotensin II blocker
C. Bendrofluazide
D. Beta-blocker
E. Frusemide

159. A 40-year-old woman complains of fever and cough. CXR reveals bilateral hilar lymphadenopathy. She also has painful nodules in her lower legs.

What is the SINGLE most *likely diagnosis*?

A. Lyme disease
B. *Mycoplasma* pneumonia
C. Sarcoidosis
D. SLE
E. Tuberculosis

160. A mother reports that her child walks upstairs one foot per step and downstairs with two feet on each step.

What age is this child?

A. I year
B. 18 months
C. 2 years
D. 3 years
E. 4 years

161. A 60-year-old woman complains of a painless but itchy rash on the outer side of her lower leg.

What is the SINGLE most *likely diagnosis*?

A. Bowen's disease
B. Discoid eczema
C. Necrobiasis lipoidica
D. Scabies
E. Tinea corporis

162. A 30-year-old woman complains of fever, headache, and painful calves. She reports that she just got back from holiday in India and she had been swimming in the sea. On examination, the conjunctivae are injected and skin changes of jaundice and purpura are noted.

What is the SINGLE most *likely diagnosis*?

A. Giardiasis
B. Leishmaniasis
C. Leptospirosis
D. Q fever
E. Relapsing fever

163. A 50-year-old man post CABG develops ventricular fibrillation while on a lignocaine drip. He does not respond to DC cardioversion. BP is 80/40. No pulse is palpable.

What is the SINGLE most *appropriate management*?

A. Administer adrenaline
B. Administer atropine
C. Needle pericardiocentesis
D. Open the chest, suction and massage the heart
E. Perform CPR

164. A 20-year-old woman presents with a neck lump. On examination, the lump lies beneath the anterior border of the sternomastoid.

What is the SINGLE most *likely diagnosis*?

A. Branchial cyst
B. Cervical lymph node
C. Goitre
D. Submandibular lymph node
E. Thyroglossal cyst

165. A 25-year-old woman presents with a midline neck lump that moves on protrusion of the tongue.

What is the SINGLE most *likely diagnosis*?

A. Branchial cyst
B. Cervical lymph node
C. Goitre
D. Submandibular lymph node
E. Thyroglossal cyst

166. A 50-year-old man who has had mastoid surgery now presents with diminished right-sided hearing. Weber lateralises to the right, and the Rinne test is negative on the right.

What is the SINGLE most *likely diagnosis*?

A. Otitis media
B. Otitis externa
C. Otosclerosis
D. Tympanic membrane perforation
E. Wax impaction

167. A 55-year-old man with hypertension is commenced on medication. Blood tests 2 weeks later show a creatinine level of 500 μmol/l.

What is the SINGLE most *likely culprit*?

A. Atenolol
B. Bendrofluazide
C. Frusemide
D. Losartan
E. Perindopril

168. A 50-year-old man complains of heel pain. It is worse when first getting out of bed. On examination, the sole of the foot is tender 3 cm superior to the heel.

What is the SINGLE most *likely diagnosis*?

A. Calcaneal apophysitis
B. Metatarsalgia
C. Plantar fasciitis
D. Reiter's disease
E. Stress fracture

169. A 20-year-old female athlete complains of right knee pain. She states it is worse when using stairs or getting up from a chair. She hears her knee grind. On examination, when the patella is pressed against the femur in an extended position, she feels pain.

What is the SINGLE most *likely diagnosis*?

A. Chondromalacia patella
B. Osgood-Schlatter disease
C. Osteochondritis dissecans
D. Meniscal tear
E. Patellar tendonitis

170. A 55-year-old man complains of headache. On fundoscopic examination, there is papilloedema. BP is 220/110.

What is the SINGLE investigation most *likely to give a definitive diagnosis*?

A. CT scan of head
B. Lumbar puncture
C. MRI scan
D. Slit lamp exam with intraocular pressure reading
E. Skull x-ray

171. A 6-year-old girl is brought in by her mother holding her right arm by her side. The child had fallen while holding her mother's hand. Flexion of the elbow causes pain. However gentle movement of the wrist is painless.

What is the SINGLE most *appropriate management*?

A. Manipulation without analgesia
B. Manipulation under IV sedation
C. Manipulation under general anaesthesia
D. Send her home with her arm in a sling
E. X-ray to show dislocation of elbow

172. A football goalkeeper complains of pain in his left forearm. He sustained a direct blow to his forearm warding off a football.

What is the SINGLE most *likely radiographic appearance of the fracture?*

A. Fracture of both the radius and ulnar
B. Fracture of the radial neck
C. Fracture of the ulnar shaft
D. Galeazzi fracture–dislocation
E. Monteggia fracture–dislocation

173. A 10-year-old boy complains of pain in his left shoulder and holds his left arm with his right arm. He fell on an extended and outstretched hand while running. On examination, there is a painful lump seen with decreased range of movement of the left shoulder.

What is the SINGLE most *appropriate treatment?*

A. Broad arm sling and analgesia
B. Collar and cuff sling
C. Initial rest and analgesia followed by manipulation
D. Manipulation under general anaesthesia
E. Open reduction and internal fixation

174. An 8-year-old boy falls off a monkey bar climbing frame. He now complains of severe right shoulder pain. There is marked bruising and swelling. You suspect a fracture of the proximal humerus.

What is the SINGLE most *common type of proximal humeral fracture in this patient?*

A. Fracture of the anatomical neck
B. Fracture of the greater tuberosity
C. Fracture of the lesser tuberosity
D. Fracture separation of the proximal humeral epiphysis
E. Greenstick fractures of the surgical neck

175. A 12-year-old boy is brought in by his mother for fever, vomiting and diarrhoea. On examination, the abdomen is soft with hyperactive bowel sounds. His sister is also unwell.

What is the SINGLE most *likely diagnosis*?

A. Acute appendicitis
B. Acute gastroenteritis
C. Cyclical vomiting syndrome
D. Inflammatory bowel disease
E. Irritable bowel syndrome

176. A 50-year-old man was commenced on an antihypertensive and is now in renal failure with a K of 2 mmol/l.

What is the SINGLE most *likely culprit*?

A. Amlodipine
B. Bendrofluazide
C. Losartan
D. Perindopril
E. Spironolactone

177. A 55-year-old woman presents with tachycardia, sweating and on examination has a displaced trachea, stridor and a positive Pemberton's sign (facial congestion when the arms are raised above her head).

What is the SINGLE most *likely diagnosis*?

A. Angioneurotic oedema
B. Epiglottitis
C. Pneumothorax
D. Retrosternal goitre
E. Subcutaneous emphysema

178. A 20-year-old man is brought into Casualty bleeding from slashed wrists. On exam, BP is 130/60, P 90. He is alert.

What is the SINGLE next *appropriate course of action*?

A. Apply dressing to wound
B. Apply external pressure to wounds
C. Gain IV access and administer blood transfusion
D. Gain IV access and start IV fluids
E. Give 100% oxygen by face mask

179. A 70-year-old woman is brought into Casualty by ambulance with profuse epistaxis. Blood is pouring from both nostrils and her mouth. She is alert and apologises for the trouble she has caused. BP is 100/60, P 110, RR 20.

What is the SINGLE next *appropriate course of action*?

A. Gain IV access and administer blood transfusion
B. Gain IV access and commence IV fluids
C. Give 100% oxygen by face mask
D. Give paracetamol, nifedipine and valium
E. Insert 8 cm Merocel nasal pack

180. A 20-year-old tall college student presents with marked SOB. He has recently returned from Nigeria. On examination, the trachea is deviated to the right, the neck veins are distended, the left lung is hyperresonant with diminished tactile vocal fremitus and there are no breath sounds. His BP is 90/50 and P 120.

What is the SINGLE most *definitive course of action*?

A. Administer 100% oxygen by face mask
B. Gain IV access and commence IV fluids
C. Insert a chest tube
D. Needle thoracostomy into the second intercostal space
E. Obtain an urgent CXR

181. A 40-year-old man involved in an RTA on the motorway presents in shock. On examination, the trachea is deviated to the right. A CXR reveals a widened mediastinum and fracture of the left first rib.

What is the SINGLE most *likely diagnosis*?

A. Aortic rupture
B. Cardiac tamponade
C. Haemothorax
D. Splenic rupture
E. Tension pneumothorax

182. A 55-year-old man complains of severe flank pain. He is writhing in discomfort. He describes the pain as starting in the right side of his back and travelling round the front down to his groin.

What is the SINGLE most *appropriate next course of action*?

A. Administer diclofenac sodium 75 mg IM
B. Arrange KUB
C. MSU for culture and sensitivities
D. Take blood for urea/lytes, calcium and uric acid
E. Urine dipstick for blood

183. A 55-year-old man with multiple sclerosis presents with urinary retention and worsening urea and creatinine levels. On examination, the bladder is palpable. He reports that he has had intermittent urinary catheterisation in the past.

What is the SINGLE most *likely diagnosis*?

A. Benign prostatic hypertrophy
B. Renal calculus
C. Retroperitoneal fibrosis
D. Urethral stricture
E. UTI

184. A 6/40 pregnant woman presents with right-sided pelvic pain. She has not had a scan for this pregnancy. There is no PV bleed. She presents to Casualty at 2 a.m. with a BP of 100/60 and P 80.

What is the SINGLE most *appropriate management*?

A. Give her a form for an outpatient ultrasound
B. Refer her to the gynae. SHO on call
C. Keep her in A&E for observation
D. Take HVS and endocervical swabs
E. Tell her to return at 9 a.m. to the Early Pregnancy Unit for a scan

185. A 60-year-old man has unstable angina and a positive exercise stress test.

What is the SINGLE most *appropriate management*?

A. Arrange coronary angiogram
B. Arrange echocardiogram
C. Fit Holter ECG
D. Waiting list for CABG
E. Waiting list for PTCA

186. A 45-year-old woman presents with palpitations and skipped heart beats at rest. Her mother had an MI at age 50. 24-hour Holter monitoring shows occasional PVCs only.

What is the SINGLE most *appropriate next course of action*?

A. Arrange coronary angiogram
B. Arrange echocardiogram
C. Arrange exercise stress test
D. Commence propranolol
E. Give reassurance

187. A patient experiences dystocia (difficult and prolonged labour) with a breech baby. Her baby weighs 9 lb but does not move his right arm.

What is the SINGLE most *likely diagnosis*?

A. Clavicle fracture
B. Fracture of shaft of humerus
C. Fracture of surgical neck of humerus
D. Pulled elbow
E. Shoulder dislocation

188. A 30-year-old man complains of double vision and droopy eyelids at the end of the day. He is a banker and sits in front of a VDU screen for 12 hours a day. You ask him to count to 50, and his voice weakens at 40.

What is the SINGLE most *likely diagnosis*?

A. Brain tumour
B. Depression
C. Multiple sclerosis
D. Myasthenia gravis
E. Polymyalgia rheumatica

189. A pure tone audiogram shows a bilateral conductive hearing loss. On examination, the patient has normal tympanic membranes.

What is the SINGLE most *likely diagnosis*?

A. Acoustic neuroma
B. Barotrauma
C. Ménière's disease
D. Otitis media with effusion
E. Otosclerosis

190. A pure tone audiogram shows bilateral high-frequency sensorineural hearing loss. The patient reports that the hearing loss has been gradual and he can't hear his wife clearly.

What is the SINGLE most *likely diagnosis?*

A. Acoustic neuroma
B. Eustachian tube dysfunction
C. Noise-induced hearing loss
D. Otosclerosis
E. Presbyacusis

191. A 20-year-old schoolteacher presents with right-sided hearing loss. Pure tone audiogram confirms a right-sided high-frequency sensorineural hearing loss.

What is the SINGLE most *likely diagnosis?*

A. Acoustic neuroma
B. Ménière's disease
C. Mumps
D. Otitis media with effusion
E. Presbyacusis

192. A range in which the true value lies.

What is the SINGLE best *term for this definition?*

A. Confidence interval
B. Forest plot
C. Median
D. Mode
E. Sensitivity

193. To determine the difference between actual and expected number of reactions.

What is the SINGLE best *statistical test?*

A. Chi-square
B. Fisher's test
C. Mann-Whitney U test
D. *P* value
E. Student's *t* test

194. The ability of a test to pick up disease.

What is the SINGLE best *term for this definition*?

A. Negative predictive value
B. Positive predictive value
C. *P* value
D. Sensitivity
E. Specificity

195. A 12-year-old girl presents with a crusty yellow patchy rash on her face, leaking golden fluid.

What is the SINGLE most *likely diagnosis*?

A. Cellulitis
B. Discoid eczema
C. Herpes zoster
D. Impetigo
E. Ringworm

196. A 22-year-old schizophrenic is unreliable with taking medication but reliable with attending community psychiatric clinic appointments.

What is the SINGLE most *appropriate management*?

A. Arrange daily visit by CPN to administer oral antipsychotics
B. Counselling
C. Depot injection
D. Detention
E. ECT

197. A 16-year-old girl presents with SOB. She has a history of asthma. She is wheezing and her chest is tight. She is unable to speak.

What is the SINGLE most *appropriate management*?

A. Administer IM adrenaline
B. Advise to take additional puffs of her short-acting β2 agonist
C. Call 999
D. Endotracheal intubation
E. Nebulised β2 agonist by face mask

198. A 40-year-old alcoholic indigent male is brought to A&E for unruliness. He is agitated, diaphoretic and then loses consciousness. There are no signs of trauma and his pupils are equal and reactive. There is a strong odour of alcohol on him and an empty bottle of whiskey.

What is the SINGLE most *likely diagnosis*?

A. Alcohol intoxication
B. Epilepsy
C. Heart block
D. Hypoglycaemia
E. Subdural haematoma

199. A 30-year-old man complains of swollen, red right knee with pain. He has a family history of gout and was recently on holiday in Bangkok. Knee aspirate is cloudy. The ESR is raised.

What is the SINGLE most *likely diagnosis*?

A. Gout
B. Osteoarthritis
C. Pseudogout
D. Reiter's disease
E. Septic arthritis

200. A 52-year-old married woman presents with PV bleeding. She reached menopause at age 48. The cervical os is nad.

What is the SINGLE next most *appropriate investigation*?

A. Endocervical swabs and HVS
B. Pap smear
C. Refer for colposcopy and iodine staining
D. Refer for transvaginal ultrasound
E. Take blood for FSH levels.

201. A 30-year-old man presents with unilateral sensorineural hearing loss and tinnitus. MRI shows a large internal auditory meatus.

What is the SINGLE most *likely diagnosis*?

A. Acoustic neuroma
B. Herpes zoster oticus
C. Ménière's disease
D. Otosclerosis
E. Viral labyrinthitis

202. A 40-year-old man presents with fever, malaise, SOB, weight loss and persistent watery rhinorrhoea. On examination, he has nasal crusting and a septal perforation.

What is the SINGLE most *likely diagnosis*?

A. Allergic rhinitis
B. Nasal polyps
C. Nasal vestibulitis
D. Nasopharyngeal carcinoma
E. Wegener's granulomatosis

203. A 50-year-old smoker presents with unilateral left cheek swelling and infraorbital nerve hyperaesthesia. On examination, he is afebrile and there are no signs of tooth root infection.

What is the SINGLE most *likely diagnosis*?

A. Acute maxillary sinusitis
B. Dacrocystitis
C. Haemophilus cellulitis
D. Maxillary antral carcinoma
E. Mumps

204. A 75-year-old woman presents with profuse epistaxis that does not respond to pressure. She denies use of aspirin, NSAIDs, or warfarin. She denies trauma.

What is the SINGLE most *likely cause of her nosebleed*?

A. Atherosclerosis
B. Coagulopathy
C. Nasal vestibulitis
D. Septal perforation
E. Sinonasal tumour

205. A 40-year-old female with diagnosed breast cancer now complains of polydipsia, polyuria, constipation and myalgia.

What is the SINGLE most *useful investigation*?

A. Bone scan
B. CT scan chest and abdomen
C. Fasting blood glucose
D. MRI pituitary gland
E. Serum calcium

206. A 4-year-old boy presents with right-sided purulent nasal discharge.

What is the SINGLE most *likely diagnosis*?

A. Bronchiectasis
B. Inhaled foreign body
C. Nasal vestibulitis
D. Rhinosinusitis
E. Sinonasal tumour

207. A 60-year-old man post TKR (total knee replacement) presents with fever, SOB and chest pain. ABG shows low paO_2 and low pCO_2.

What is the SINGLE most *likely diagnosis*?

A. Atelectasis
B. Myocardial infarction
C. Pneumonia
D. Pulmonary embolism
E. Pulmonary oedema

208. A 90-year-old woman presents with an irregular pulse with rate of 130.

What is the SINGLE most *useful treatment*?

A. Aspirin and digoxin
B. Atenolol
C. Heparin and digoxin
D. Lignocaine
E. Warfarin and digoxin

209. A 50-year-old man presents with a persistently elevated BP of 170/120 and a potassium level of 3 mmol/l. He also reports nocturia. He is not on any medication.

What is the SINGLE most *likely diagnosis*?

A. Conn's syndrome
B. Cushing's syndrome
C. Hypercalcaemia
D. Phaeochromocytoma
E. Polycystic kidney disease

210. A 40-year-old woman is found to have both iron and folate deficiency on routine blood tests. She also reports that her stools are difficult to flush.

What is the SINGLE most *useful advice*?

A. Gluten-free diet
B. Lactose-free diet
C. Low-fat diet
D. More spinach and red meat
E. Take multivitamins.

211. A 4-year-old boy accidentally swallowed some tablets. On examination, pupils are pinpoint and respirations are shallow with marked hypotonia.

What is the SINGLE most *likely diagnosis*?

A. Atropine poisoning
B. Benzodiazepine poisoning
C. Opiate poisoning
D. Paracetamol poisoning
E. Tricyclic antidepressant poisoning

212. A 7-year-old boy with ADHD on a norepinephrine reuptake inhibitor attempts suicide.

What is the SINGLE most *likely diagnosis*?

A. Concomitant depression
B. Concomitant paranoid-schizophrenia
C. Personality disorder
D. Side effect of norepinephrine reuptake inhibitor
E. Sign of sexual abuse

213. A 20-year-old salesman complains of episodes of perioral tingling and tingling in his fingertips for the past 2 months since he started working in a new office.

What is the SINGLE most *likely diagnosis*?

A. Excessive caffeine intake
B. Hypocalcaemia
C. Hypoglycaemia
D. Panic attack
E. Spider venom

214. A 30-year-old man is stabbed in the left chest with a BBQ skewer. He was haemodynamically stable on arrival to A&E and then suddenly has a drop in BP to 60/40 with a thready pulse.

What is the SINGLE most *likely diagnosis*?

A. Cardiac tamponade
B. Haemothorax
C. Myocardial infarction
D. Ruptured ascending aorta
E. Tension pneumothorax

215. A 20-year-old woman with bipolar disorder is commenced on lithium.

What SINGLE blood *test should you be monitoring besides lithium levels*?

A. Calcium
B. Clotting factors
C. Full blood count
D. Thyroid function test
E. Urea and electrolytes

216. A 30-year-old schizophrenic has been on treatment for 1 year but now complains of a dry mouth, gynaecomastia, impotence and restlessness.

What is the SINGLE most *likely cause*?

A. Amitryptiline
B. Chlorpromazine
C. Lithium
D. Sodium valproate
E. Venlafaxine

217. A 65-year-old farmer states that he is having trouble sleeping and is forgetful. He is in debt and has recently been bereaved.

What is the SINGLE most *likely diagnosis*?

A. Anxiety
B. Delirium
C. Dementia
D. Depression
E. Insomnia

218. A 16-year-old girl requests contraception. She has been seeing her 17-year-old steady boyfriend for 1 month and would
like to become intimate.

What is the SINGLE most *appropriate form of contraception?*

A. Condoms
B. Depoprovera injection
C. Microgynon
D. Norethisterone
E. Oestrogen implant

219. A 40-year-old married woman requests contraception. She
has always had heavy painful periods. She has 3 children. She
is needle-phobic and has a busy schedule.

What is the SINGLE most *appropriate form of contraception?*

A. Diaphragm
B. IUCD
C. Microgynon
D. Mirena coil
E. Oestrogen implant

220. A 35-year-old heavy smoker on anti-epileptic drugs requests
contraception.

What is the SINGLE most *appropriate form of contraception?*

A. Condoms
B. Depoprovera every 10 weeks
C. Diaphragm
D. Norethisterone
E. Norplant

221. A 6-week-old baby is diagnosed with pyloric stenosis.

What is the SINGLE most *likely electrolyte disturbance?*

A. Hypokalaemia
B. Metabolic acidosis
C. Metabolic alkalosis
D. Respiratory acidosis
E. Respiratory alkalosis

222. A 22-year-old asthmatic comes for her review and reports that she still wheezes despite being on salbutamol and beclomethasone. PEF is 70% predicted.

What is the SINGLE most *appropriate medication*?

A. Add LABA
B. Add I week of prednisolone
C. Double the steroid dosage
D. Nebulised salbutamol treatment
E. Oral theophylline

223. A 19-year-old female on Microgynon presents with PV bleeding after intercourse. She has a long-term partner and no other symptoms.

What is the SINGLE most *likely cause*?

A. Breakthrough bleeding
B. Cervical carcinoma
C. Cervical ectropion
D. Cervical polyp
E. *Chlamydia* infection

224. A 30-year-old woman complains of 7 months of amenorrhoea, facial hair and acne. She has put on a stone in the past month.

What is the SINGLE most *likely diagnosis*?

A. Adrenal tumour
B. Cushing's disease
C. Idiopathic
D. Ovarian carcinoma
E. Polycystic ovarian disease

225 A 60-year-old man with inoperable obstructive oesophageal carcinoma requires feeding.

What is the SINGLE most *appropriate method of feeding*?

A. Ensure liquid feeds
B. NG feeding tube
C. IV fluids
D. Percutaneous endoscopic gastrostomy
E. Total parenteral nutrition

226. A 40-year-old man has intractable hiccups.

What is the SINGLE most *appropriate medication from the list below*?

A. Amantadine
B. Anti-psychotic (chlorpromazine or haloperidol)
C. Benzodiazepine (diazepam)
D. Cinnarazine
E. Corticosteroid (prednisolone)

227. A 25-year-old woman on the pill presents with profuse BRBPR. Barium enema shows extensive thumb-printing involving the entire colon.

What is the SINGLE most *likely diagnosis*?

A. Colon carcinoma
B. Crohn's disease
C. Diverticulitis
D. Ischaemic colitis
E. Ulcerative colitis

228. A 70-year-old frail woman complains of a dragging sensation down below. On examination, there is a second-degree uterine prolapse.

What is the SINGLE most *appropriate management*?

A. Do nothing.
B. Elevest laparoscopic procedure of shortening the ligaments
C. Pelvic floor exercises
D. Ring pessary
E. Vaginal hysterectomy

229. A 40-year-old obese pregnant woman is about to embark on a transatlantic flight. Her grandmother had a DVT at age 50.

What is the SINGLE most *appropriate management*?

A. Advise her that she cannot fly during pregnancy as she is of too high risk
B. Advise her to fly first-class to ensure plenty of leg room
C. Advise her to take aspirin pre-boarding and every 4–6 hours during the flight.
D. Advise her to wear graduated compression stockings
E. Reassure her that she will be fine

230. A 35-year-old NIDDM female presents with a large goitre. Histologically thyroid tissue is replaced by lymphoid tissue.

What is the SINGLE most *likely diagnosis*?

A. Anaplastic thyroid carcinoma
B. Follicular thyroid carcinoma
C. Hashimoto's thyroiditis
D. Medullary thyroid carcinoma
E. Papillary thyroid carcinoma

231. A 25-year-old female was exposed to radiation in Russia and is diagnosed with thyroid carcinoma.

What is the SINGLE most *common form of thyroid carcinoma*?

A. Anaplastic thyroid carcinoma
B. Follicular thyroid carcinoma
C. Medullary thyroid carcinoma
D. Mixed follicular/papillary thyroid carcinoma
E. Papillary thyroid carcinoma

232. You are preparing a patient for total thyroidectomy.

What is the SINGLE most *important pre-operative management*?

A. Check ABG
B. Check clotting factors
C. Check TFTs
D. Give SC heparin
E. Refer to ENT to check the integrity of the recurrent laryngeal nerve.

233. In which thyroid condition will an FNAC not be adequate and a tissue biopsy be more preferable?

What is the SINGLE *best answer*?

A. Anaplastic carcinoma
B. Follicular cell carcinoma
C. Medullary carcinoma
D. Mixed follicular/papillary carcinoma
E. Papillary carcinoma

234. A 25-year-old male presents with a painless testicular swelling and complains of a pulling sensation in his groin. He has a history of undescended testes.

What is the SINGLE most *appropriate next investigation*?

A. Alpha-fetoprotein, β-HCG, LDH
B. CT scan of abdomen
C. FNAC
D. Tissue biopsy
E. Ultrasound

235. A 40-year-old woman diagnosed with breast cancer has undergone both radiotherapy and chemotherapy and now presents with right femur pain. She denies trauma.

What is the SINGLE most *likely diagnosis*?

A. Bone metastasis
B. Hypercalcaemia
C. Osteomalacia
D. Osteoporosis
E. Pathological fracture

236. What is the SINGLE most *appropriate management* for this patient?

A. Calcichew forte
B. Combination chemotherapy
C. Intramedullary nail fixation
D. IV bisphosphonates
E. Radiotherapy

237. A 50-year-old man on digoxin now complains of abdominal pain and muscle weakness. ECG shows peak T waves and ST segment depression.

What is the SINGLE most *appropriate management*?

A. Dialysis
B. FAB fragments of digoxin-specific antibodies
C. IV 10% calcium gluconate
D. IV dextrose and insulin
E. Nebulised salbutamol

238. A 40-year-old woman attends for a pap smear. On speculum exam, a small, smooth, rounded lump is noted on her cervix. She has no symptoms.

What is the SINGLE most *likely diagnosis*?

A. Cervical carcinoma
B. Cervical ectropion
C. Cervical polyp
D. Cervical wart
E. Nabothian cyst

239. A Nigerian mother brings in her 15-month-old for the MMR vaccine. She informs you that she and her baby have HIV.

What is the SINGLE most *appropriate course of action*?

A. Administer MMR
B. Administer single MMR vaccines
C. Delay MMR vaccine
D. Give inactivated vaccine
E. Refuse to administer MMR

240. A 65-year-old woman presents with a unilateral painful rash across her torso. On examination, there are crusts and vesicles. She states that her former GP had given her antiviral medication but that she is still in intense pain. She takes digoxin.

What is the SINGLE most *appropriate medication*?

A. Advise her to continue acyclovir for another week
B. Amantadine
C. Amitriptyline
D. Carbamazepine
E. Gabapentin

241. A 9-year-old Native American girl presents with fever, malaise, painful throat, trismus and is drooling saliva. On exam, temperature is 40°C and there is a white membrane covering the entire left tonsil.

What is the SINGLE investigation most *likely to give a definitive diagnosis*?

A. EBV serology (anti-EBNA I IgG)
B. Full blood count
C. Microlatex test for diphtheria anti-toxin
D. Monospot test
E. Throat swab for culture

242. A 40-year-old surgeon states that he was tested by occupational health and was informed that he was a hepatitis B carrier. He requests testing to determine whether he may operate.

What is the SINGLE most *appropriate investigation*?

A. Hep BsAb
B. Hep BsAg
C. Hep BeAb
D. Hep BeAg
E. Hep BcAg

243. A 30-year-old homosexual male reports that he recently had unprotected sex with a man who has just informed him that he is HIV positive. He now asks you what the latest time he can take post-exposure prophylaxis.

What is the SINGLE *best answer*?

A. 2 hours
B. 12 hours
C. 24 hours
D. 48 hours
E. 72 hours

244. A 30-year-old pregnant woman presents with vesicles along the length of her right arm.

What is the SINGLE investigation most *likely to provide a definitive diagnosis*?

A. Direct immunofluorescence with fluorescent-tagged antibody
B. ESR
C. Skin biopsy
D. Tzanck smear
E. Wound swab for culture

245. What is the SINGLE best *treatment for this patient*?

A. Acyclovir
B. Capsaicin cream
C. Corticosteroids
D. Flucloxacillin
E. VZV vaccination

246. A 45-year-old woman reports a green discharge from her right nipple. She is concerned. On exam, there are no lumps and no axillary lymphadenopathy. There is redness and tenderness around the nipple.

What is the SINGLE most *likely diagnosis*?

A. Breast abscess
B. Duct ectasia
C. Intraductal papilloma
D. Mastitis
E. Paget's disease

247. A 25-year-old Afro-Carribean woman is concerned, as she has felt a hard lump in her right breast. She describes it as a marble in her breast. She denies trauma. On exam, a single mobile firm 1 cm lump is palpable. There are no axillary lymph nodes, no skin changes and no nipple discharge.

What is the SINGLE most *likely diagnosis*?

A. Breast abscess
B. Breast carcinoma
C. Fat necrosis
D. Fibroadenoma
E. Fibrocystic disease

248. A 43-year-old woman presents with a lump. The lump is located anteroinferior to the external auditory meatus and inferior to the zygomatic arch. It is smooth and painless. She reports that it has been present for 1 year.

What is the SINGLE most *likely diagnosis*?

A. Mumps
B. Pancoast tumour
C. Parotitis
D. Pleomorphic parotid adenoma
E. Preauricular lymph node

249. A 50-year-old smoker presents with left-sided shoulder pain and weakness, and paraesthesiae in his left arm and hand. On examination, miosis and ptosis are also present.

What is the SINGLE most *likely diagnosis*?

A. Brachial plexus palsy
B. Frozen shoulder
C. Pancoast tumour
D. Superior vena cava syndrome
E. TIA

250. A 55-year-old businessman from Hong Kong presents with severe epigastric pain, worse during the day. He reports that he vomits after eating food. He denies weight loss. On examination there is mild epigastric tenderness.

What is the SINGLE most *likely diagnosis*?

A. Duodenal ulcer
B. Gastric ulcer
C. GERD
D. Mallory-Weiss tear
E. Stomach carcinoma

251. A 10-year-old boy with cystic fibrosis presents with fever and cough. CXR reveals pneumatocoeles.

What is the SINGLE most *likely organism*?

A. *Haemophilus influenzae*
B. *Mycobacterium tuberculosis*
C. *Pseudomonas aeruginosa*
D. *Staphylococcus aureus*
E. *Streptococcus pneumoniae*

252. A 50-year-old alcoholic male complains of currant-jelly-coloured sputum. CXR reveals upper lobe consolidation with a bowing fissure.

What is the SINGLE most *likely organism*?

A. *Klebsiella pneumoniae*
B. *Mycobacterium tuberculosis*
C. *Pseudomonas aeruginosa*
D. *Staphylococcus aureus*
E. *Streptococcus pneumoniae*

253. A 55-year-old man postoperatively is noted to have tachy-cardia, tachypnoea, oliguria and warm extremities. Mean BP is 40 mmHg. Pulmonary artery wedge pressure reads 17 mmHg.

What is the SINGLE most *appropriate treatment*?

A. Antibodies to tumour necrosis factor
B. Dobutamine
C. Dopamine
D. Mannitol
E. Norepinephrine

254. A 16-year-old girl is brought into Casualty unconscious. T = 40°C. ECG shows peak T waves. Her friends report that she took an illicit drug but do not know which one.

What is the SINGLE most *likely poison*?

A. Amphetamines
B. Cocaine
C. LSD
D. Marijuana
E. MDMA (ecstasy)

255. A neonate develops jaundice 6 hours after delivery. The neonate has a positive direct Coombs test and the bilirubin is 150 mmol/l with a haematocrit of 48%.

What is the SINGLE most *likely diagnosis*?

A. Biliary atresia
B. Breast milk jaundice
C. Galactosaemia
D. Haemolytic disease of the newborn
E. Hepatitis C

256. A 20-year-old motorcyclist is involved in an RTA. On exam-ination, there is blood present at the urethral meatus, the bladder is palpable at the umbilicus and a high-riding prostate is palpable on PR. The man is agitated and explains that he cannot void.

What is the SINGLE next most *appropriate intervention*?

A. Ascending urethrogram
B. IVU
C. 16F Foley urethral catheterisation
D. Retrograde urethrogram
E. Suprapubic catheterisation

257. A 30-year-old 30/40 pregnant woman is involved in an RTA.

What is the SINGLE special *precaution to take with this woman during the initial assessment*?

A. Administer IV fluids only when she is haemodynamically unstable
B. Administer Rhesus immunoglobulin therapy
C. Avoid pelvic x-rays
D. Transport her in the left lateral decubitus position with her right leg raised
E. Transport her in the right lateral decubitus position with her left leg raised

258. A 60-year-old army sargeant reports gradual right-sided hearing loss. Pure tone audiogram shows a dip at 4 kHz.

What is the SINGLE most *likely diagnosis*?

A. Acoustic neuroma
B. Noise-induced hearing loss
C. Otitis media with effusion
D. Otosclerosis
E. Presbyacusis

259. A 35-year-old man states that he feels a lump in his throat that does not enable him to swallow foods or liquids. He is not drooling saliva. He has no associated weight loss.

What is the SINGLE most *likely diagnosis*?

A. Achalasia
B. GERD
C. Globus hystericus
D. Oesophagitis
E. Pharyngeal pouch

260. A 30-year-old man is assaulted and battered. On examination, there is bruising around the left 12th rib in his back. He has frank haematuria.

What is the SINGLE most *appropriate initial investigation*?

A. Arteriography
B. CT scan
C. Excretory urogram
D. IV pyelogram
E. Ultrasound

261. A 30-year-old woman complains of aphthous ulcers, diarrhoea, fatigue and weight loss. On examination, there is both angular stomatitis and glossitis.

What is the SINGLE most *likely diagnosis?*

A. Crohn's disease
B. Coeliac disease
C. Irritable bowel disease
D. Malabsorption
E. Ulcerative colitis

262. A 55-year-old woman complains of severe chest pain. On arrival to Casualty, she becomes drowsy. Her BP is now 80/55 mmHg with a pulse rate of 45. An ECG shows first-degree heart block.

What is the SINGLE next most *appropriate management?*

A. Atropine IV
B. Epinephrine IV
C. Lignocaine IV
D. Propranolol
E. Transcutaneous pacing patches

263. A 50-year-old man 2 days post MI is now found unconscious with pulseless electrical activity.

What is the SINGLE most appropriate *resuscitative drug treatment while assessing for cause?*

A. Adrenaline (epinephrine)
B. Atropine
C. Lignocaine
D. Propranolol
E. Verapamil

264. A 55-year-old woman complains of hearing loss, pulsatile tinnitis and hoarseness. On examination, a reddish-blue pulsatile mass is seen behind the tympanic membrane

What is the SINGLE most *likely diagnosis?*

A. Aberrant intrapetrous internal carotid artery
B. Cholesteatoma
C. Glomus jugulare tumour
D. Histiocytosis X
E. Prominent jugular bulb

265. A newborn is noted to have a large midline neck swelling involving the tongue. The mass is soft and transilluminates.

What is the SINGLE most *likely diagnosis*?

A. Branchial cyst
B. Cervical lymph node
C. Cystic hygroma
D. Goitre
E. Thyroglossal cyst

266. A 30-year-old DIY enthusiast reports that he was drilling a metal sheet and now has intense pain in his right eye.

What is the SINGLE most *appropriate management*?

A. Arrange for x-ray to exclude metallic foreign body
B. Irrigate eye with 1 L of saline
C. Measure intraocular pressures
D. Perform fluorescein dye test for corneal abrasion
E. Refer urgently to ophthalmologist on call

267. A 10-year-old boy is given amoxicillin for otitis media. He presents in anaphylactic shock. His mother was not aware that amoxicillin was in the same class as penicillin and had not informed the doctor that the child was allergic to penicillin.

What is the SINGLE most *appropriate initial treatment*?

A. IM 1:5000 adrenaline 500 mcg or 0.1 ml
B. IM 1:1000 adrenaline 250 mcg or 0.25 ml
C. IM 1:1000 adrenaline 500 mcg or 0.5 ml
D. IV 1:10,000 adrenaline 250 mcg
E. IV 1:1000 adrenaline 500 mcg or 0.5 ml

268. A 6-year-old girl comes in with a bead stuck in her right ear. She is co-operative.

What is the SINGLE most *appropriate management*?

A. Hook
B. Magnet
C. Microsuction to remove under microscope
D. Syringing
E. Removal under GA

269. A 2-year-old boy comes in with an insect in his left ear. He is distressed.

What is the SINGLE next most *appropriate management*?

A. Hook
B. Instill mineral oil or lignocaine 2%
C. Irrigate with waterpik
D. Magnet
E. Remove with alligator forceps

270. A 2-year-old girl presents with a pea in her right ear. She is not co-operative and screams when you approach her.

What is the SINGLE most *appropriate management*?

A. Book for removal under GA
B. Hook
C. Microsuction using microscope (ENT)
D. Remove with forceps
E. Syringing

271. What is the SINGLE best *guidance for basic life support CPR*?

A. Place interlocked hands on lower sternum and carry out chest compressions to ventilation ratio of 5:1
B. Place interlocked hands on mid-sternum and carry out chest compressions to ventilation ratio of 5:1
C. Place interlocked hands on lower sternum and carry out chest compressions to ventilation ratio of 15:2
D. Place interlocked hands on mid-sternum and carry out chest compressions to ventilation ratio of 15:2
E. Place interlocked hands on lower sternum and carry out chest compressions to ventilation ratio of 5:2

272. A US sheep farmer presents with a crusty blister inside his nostril.

What is the SINGLE most *likely diagnosis*?

A. Bacillus anthracis
B. Cryptosporidiosis
C. Orf disease (parapoxvirus)
D. Q-fever (*Coxiella burnetii*)
E. Wegener's granulomatosis

273. A 50-year-old man with fungating malignant melanoma on his back requests medication.

What is the SINGLE most *appropriate treatment*?

A. Capsaicin cream
B. Fusidic acid cream
C. Metronidazole gel
D. Neomycin ointment
E. Terbinafine cream

274. A 35-year-old woman has 3 spontaneous abortions in her second trimester of pregnancy. On exam, she has a discoid rash, photosensitivity and digital cyanosis. Blood tests reveal a positive Coombs test and autoimmune thrombocytopenia.

What is the SINGLE most *likely diagnosis*?

A. Antiphospholipid syndrome
B. Chlamydial infection
C. Endometriosis
D. Septate uterus
E. Trisomy 16

275. What is the SINGLE investigation in this patient *most likely to provide a definitive diagnosis*?

A. Chromosomal testing
B. Endocervical and HVS swabs
C. Gynaecologic laparoscopy
D. Lupus anticoagulant + anticardiolipin IgG antibodies
E. Transvaginal ultrasound

276. A 70-year-old female presents unconscious with pinpoint pupils and respiratory depression. Her husband reports an empty box of coproxamol at home by the bedside.

What is the SINGLE most *appropriate treatment*?

A. Acetylcysteine
B. Activated charcoal po
C. Diazepam IV
D. Flumazenil
E. Naloxone IV

277. A 40-year-old man complains of bone pain in his thigh and headaches. On examination, the skull is enlarged and hearing loss is noted. X ray of the femur shows both osteolytic and sclerotic changes.

What is the SINGLE most *likely diagnosis*?

A. Osteomalacia
B. Osteoporosis
C. Osteosarcoma
D. Paget's disease
E. Pituitary tumour

278. What is the SINGLE most *useful treatment for this patient*? (Same patient as question 277)

A. Calcichew forte
B. Cox-2 inhibitors
C. IV pamidronate
D. NSAIDs
E. SC injection of salmon calcitonin

279. A 40-year-old woman is fitted with a Nova T copper IUCD. The smear test taken 2 months later reports presence of bacteria.

What is the SINGLE most *likely organism*?

A. *Actinomzces*
B. *Gardnerella*
C. Human papilloma virus
D. *Neisseria gonorrhoea*
E. *Trichomonas vaginalis*

280. A 20-year-old known IDDM presents with confusion and sweating. Shortly thereafter, he loses consciousness. Fingerprick glucose is 1.5 mmol/l.

What is the SINGLE next most *appropriate treatment*?

A. Hypostop gel
B. Glucagon IM 1 mg
C. IV infusion of octreotide 30 ng/kg/minute
D. 50 ml of 20% dextrose solution IV
E. 25 ml of 50% dextrose solution IV

281. A 70-year-old man with end-stage COPD complains of copious chest secretions.

What is the SINGLE most *appropriate medication*?

A. Atropine
B. Cyclizine
C. Glycopyrronium
D. Hyoscine butylbromide
E. Hyoscine hydrobromide

282. A 25-year-old woman requests genetic testing for breast cancer. Both her mother and grandmother died in their early 50s of breast cancer.

What is the SINGLE most *appropriate management for this patient*?

A. Offer her annual breast ultrasound
B. Offer her annual mammogram
C. Reassure her that she is too young to develop breast cancer
D. Refer her to the breast screening clinic
E. Refer her for genetic testing

283. A 75-year-old woman with end-stage COPD complains of breathlessness on the ward. She is anxious.

What is the SINGLE most *appropriate management*?

A. Administer levomepromazine
B. Administer midazolam
C. Administer oramorph
D. Advise the nurse to increase the oxygen flow
E. Arrange for V/Q scan

284. A 30-year-old NIDDM female presents with axillary pain and lumps present for months. On examination, there are multiple pustules and ulcers with discharging sinuses. There is no axillary lymphadenopathy.

What is the SINGLE most *likely diagnosis*?

A. Crohn's disease
B. Furunculosis
C. Hydradenitis suppurutiva
D. Lymphogranuloma venereum
E. Scrofuloderma

285. A 25-year-old male athlete presents with a fluctuant 4 cm mass with surrounding cellulitis in his right armpit.

What is the SINGLE most *common organism*?

A. *Escherichia coli*
B. *Mycobacterium tuberculosis*
C. *Pseudomonas aeruginosa*
D. *Staphylococcus aureus*
E. *Streptococcus pyogenes*

286. A 70-year-old man presents with a punched-out ulcer between his toes. He is a heavy smoker and drinker. On examination, the ulcer is yellow in colour, and the foot turns red when dangling off the bed.

What is the SINGLE most *likely diagnosis*?

A. Arterial ischaemic ulcer
B. Malignancy
C. Neuropathic ulcer
D. Pressure ulcer
E. Venous stasis ulcer

287. A 65-year-old woman complains of a painful discharging ulcer above her ankle on the inner side of her left lower leg. On examination, the base of the ulcer is red and is covered by a yellow fibrous tissue. The border is irregular. The skin is tight and shiny.

What is the SINGLE most *likely diagnosis*?

A. Arterial ischaemic ulcer
B. Malignancy
C. Neuropathic ulcer
D. Pressure ulcer
E. Venous stasis ulcer

288. A 30-year-old man presents with deformed swollen right ankle. On examination, the posterior tibialis and dorsalis pedis arteries are not palpable.

What is the SINGLE next most *appropriate management*?

A. Arrange urgent arteriogram
B. Obtain an urgent ankle x-ray
C. Prepare the pt for EUA and reduction
D. Reduce the ankle dislocation
E. Refer urgently to the vascular team

289. A 20-year-old university student complains that there are insects burrowing and crawling under his skin (formication).

What is the SINGLE most *likely cause*?

A. Cocaine
B. Heroin
C. Marijuana
D. MDMA (ecstasy)
E. Methamphetamine

290. A 20-year-old woman with ulcerative colitis complains of acute flare-up with fever, intense abdominal pain, diarrhoea and BRBPR. She is already on maintenance treatment.

What is the SINGLE most *useful medication*?

A. Azathioprine
B. Ciprofloxacin
C. Methylprednisolone
D. Sulfasalazine
E. Tumour necrosis factor inhibitor (IV infusion)

291. A 20-year-old woman is brought into Casualty as a sudden cardiac arrest. Histopathology shows LV hypertrophy with extensive fibrosis. The myofibrillar architecture is in disarray and forms a whorled pattern.

What is the SINGLE most *likely diagnosis*?

A. Aortic stenosis
B. Idiopathic hypertrophic subaortic stenosis
C. Restrictive cardiomyopathy
D. Ruptured chordae tendonae
E. Type II glycogen storage disease

292. An 11/40 pregnant 34-year-old woman would like to be screened for Down's syndrome baby. She is adamant she wants testing now and does not want to wait.

What is the SINGLE most *appropriate screening test*?

A. Amniocentesis
B. Chorionic villus sampling
C. Nuchal translucency test
D. Percutaneous umbilical blood sampling
E. Triple blood test

293. An 11-month-old baby has stopped breathing and there is no circulation.

What is the SINGLE most appropriate *management of chest compression:rescue breaths*?

A. 5:1 at a rate of 100 compressions per minute 1 finger's width below the nipple line in the middle of the chest
B. 5:1 at a rate of 120 compressions per minute1 finger's width below the nipple line in the middle of the chest
C. 5:1 at a rate of 100 compressions per minute 2 fingers' width above the junction of the rib margin and sternum
D. 15:2 at a rate of 100 compressions per minute 1 finger's width below the nipple line in the middle of the chest
E. 15:2 at a rate of 100 compressions per minute 2 fingers' width above the junction of the rib margin and sternum

294. A 20-year-old woman complains of itchy, gritty red eyes with crusts and dandruff on her lashes.

What is the SINGLE most *likely diagnosis*?

A. Allergic conjunctivitis
B. Bacterial conjunctivitis
C. Blepharitis
D. Episcleritis
E. Viral conjunctivitis

295. A 55-year-old woman presents with left calf swelling and pain. On examination, pain is elicited on forced dorsiflexion of the foot with the knee straight.

What is the SINGLE most *appropriate initial investigation*?

A. Contrast venography
B. D-dimer levels
C. Duplex ultrasonography
D. Impedance plethysmography
E. MRI

296. A male patient undergoes genetic testing and is found to have mutations of both *BRCA1* and *BRCA2*. He asks what he is most at risk of with these mutations.

What is the SINGLE *best answer*?

A. Breast carcinoma
B. Colorectal carcinoma
C. Pancreatic carcinoma
D. Prostate carcinoma
E. Stomach carcinoma

297. He asks what the risk is of his daughter developing breast cancer. (Same patient as question 296)

What is the SINGLE *correct answer*?

A. 1:8
B. 1:4
C. 1:2
D. 1:1
E. Nil

298. A 70-year-old male with metastatic VIPoma complains of intractable diarrhoea.

What is the SINGLE most *useful medication*?

A. Ciprofloxacin
B. Codeine phosphate
C. Loperamide
D. Octreotide
E. Prednisolone

299. A 50-year-old man with rectal carcinoma complains of persistent diarrhoea.

What is the SINGLE most *likely acid–base disturbance*?

A. Metabolic acidosis
B. Metabolic alkalosis
C. Respiratory acidosis
D. Respiratory alkalosis
E. Mixed acid–base disorder

300. A 40-year-old man presents with raised alkaline phosphatase and bilirubin. He smokes 20 cigarettes a day and drinks 30 units of alcohol a week.

    What is the SINGLE most *likely cause from the list below?*

    A. Alcoholic hepatitis
    B. Bone metastasis
    C. Chronic liver disease
    D. Primary sclerosing cholangitis
    E. Viral hepatitis

301. A farmer is found dead by his neighbour. His neighbour reports seeing him spray his farm 1 month ago. Autopsy reveals mouth ulcers, pulmonary oedema, liver damage and renal failure. The conclusion is that he died of accidental poisoning.

    What is the SINGLE most *likely poison?*

    A. Arsenic
    B. Carbamate pesticide
    C. Organophosphorus pesticide
    D. Paraquat
    E. Urea pesticide

302. A 40-year-old woman with manic-depressive disorder now presents with a host of symptoms: vomiting, diarrhoea, hypothermia, weakness, confusion, and tremor.

    What is the SINGLE most *likely cause?*

    A. Fluoxetine
    B. Haloperidol
    C. Lithium
    D. Olanzapine
    E. Sodium valproate

303. A 45-year-old man presents with severe gnawing epigastric pain, weight loss and diarrhoea. On endoscopy, there are multiple gastric ulcers.

    What is the SINGLE next *most appropriate test to exclude Zollinger-Ellison syndrome?*

    A. Amylase
    B. Basal acid output
    C. Calcium
    D. Fasting gastrin
    E. Secretin stimulation test

304. A 30-year-old man on treatment for schizophrenia becomes confused with altered state of consciousness, labile BP, sweating, tachycardia and hyperthermia.

What is the SINGLE most *appropriate management*?

A. Activated charcoal
B. Administer antimuscarinic drugs
C. Administer isotonic sodium chloride
D. Cooling, bromocriptine and dantrolene
E. ECT

305. A 65-year-old man with terminal cancer presents with suspected superior vena cava obstruction. There is swelling of the face and neck and non-pulsatile dilated neck veins.

What is the SINGLE most *appropriate medication*?

A. Dexamethasone 16 mg oral/SC/IV
B. Frusemide p.o.
C. Glycopyrronium in syringe driver
D. Haloperidol 5 mg oral/SC
E. Midazolam 5–10 mg SC

306. A 60-year-old man with metastatic prostate carcinoma presents with spinal cord compression.

What is the SINGLE most *appropriate initial medication*?

A. Dexamethasone IV
B. Midazolam IV
C. Oramorph
D. Oxygen
E. Nil. Prepare for theatre

307. A 20-year-old female presents with blepharospasm and periorbital twitching. Her family says she has a fixed stare. She has a history of migraines and is on medication.

What is the SINGLE most *likely culprit*?

A. Carbamazepine
B. Cyclizine
C. Metoclopramide
D. Phencyclidine
E. Promethazine

308. A 15-year-old schoolgirl complains of period pains. She has a regular cycle.

What is the SINGLE most *appropriate management*?

A. Arrange transvaginal ultrasound
B. Prescribe mefenamic acid
C. Prescribe norethisterone
D. Prescribe tranexamic acid
E. Suggest commencing coc

309. A 40-year-old Afro-Carribean female presents with heavy and prolonged periods with flooding and passage of clots.

What is the SINGLE most *appropriate management*?

A. Arrange transvaginal ultrasound prior to medication
B. Commence coc
C. Mirena coil
D. Prescribe tranexamic acid
E. Transfuse blood

310. A 20-year-old woman presents with heavy periods. She states her periods are irregular. She has a new boyfriend. Her smear test is up-to-date and normal.

What is the SINGLE most *appropriate management*?

A. Arrange transvaginal ultrasound
B. Prescribe mefenamic acid
C. Prescribe norethisterone
D. Prescribe tranexamic acid
E. Suggest commencing coc

311. A 70-year-old man becomes acutely confused. On examination, he has prosapagnosia (inability to identify pictures of animals or famous persons). He has involuntary writhing movement of his right hand with abnormal posturing when attempting to use his right hand. Brisk tendon jerk reflexes and plantar extensor are present on the right.

What is the SINGLE most *likely diagnosis*?

A. Creutzfieldt-Jakob disease
B. Fronto-temporal lobar degeneration
C. Lewy body dementia
D. Multi-infarct dementia
E. Pick's disease

312. A 75-year-old woman is noted to have early loss of insight, social awareness and emotional blunting. She exhibits progressive fluent empty spontaneous speech with loss of word meaning but with preservation of anterograde memory and visuospatial skills.

What is the SINGLE most *likely diagnosis*?

A. Creutzfieldt-Jakob disease
B. Fronto-temporal lobar degeneration
C. Lewy body dementia
D. Multi-infarct dementia
E. Pick's disease

313. A 60-year-old businessman is brought in by his family as there has been a progressive change in his personality and social conduct. He is disinhibited, impulsive, irritable, apathetic, etc. with labile emotional moods (tearful). They also note that he has become more forgetful and describes nonexistent events. His speech shows signs of echolalia, perserverance and late mutism.

What is the SINGLE most *likely diagnosis*?

A. Creutzfieldt-Jakob disease
B. Fronto-temporal lobar degeneration
C. Lewy body dementia
D. Multi-infarct dementia
E. Pick's disease

314. A 30-year-old female presents with bilateral conductive hearing loss and describes paracusis willisi (an ability to hear better in a noisy environment). She states that her mother is deaf.

What is the SINGLE most *likely diagnosis*?

A. Alport syndrome
B. Neurofibromatosis
C. Osteogenesis imperfecta
D. Otosclerosis
E. Waardenburg syndrome

315. A 60-year-old woman complains of persistent thick green foul-smelling sputum tinged with blood off and on throughout the year for many years. On examination, you auscultate wheezes, rhonchi, rales and pleural rub. She also has clubbed fingers.

What is the SINGLE most *likely diagnosis*?

A. Alpha-1-antitrypsin deficiency
B. Bronchiectasis
C. Cystic fibrosis
D. Sarcoidosis
E. Tuberculosis

316. A 70-year-old female on a low-fibre (low-residue) diet complains of bright red blood per rectum and weight loss.

What is the SINGLE most *likely diagnosis*?

A. Crohn's disease
B. Colorectal carcinoma
C. Diverticular disease
D. Ischaemic colitis
E. Ulcerative colitis

317. A 20-year-old woman suffering from depression is brought to A&E after a paracetamol overdose. You need to check her paracetamol blood levels. How long after ingestion should you ideally check this?

What is the SINGLE *best answer*?

A. 2 hours
B. 3 hours
C. 4 hours
D. 6 hours
E. 12 hours

318. You receive the following arterial blood gas report: pH 7.49, pCO_2 4 kPa (40 mmHg), HCO_3 3 kPa (23 mmHg).

What is the SINGLE *best interpretation*?

A. Normal
B. Uncompensated metabolic alkalosis
C. Partially compensated metabolic alkalosis
D. Uncompensated respiratory alkalosis
E. Partially compensated respiratory alkalosis

319. You receive the following arterial blood gas report: pH 7.35, pCO_2 3.8 kPa (28 mmHg), HCO_3 2 kPA (15 mmHg).

What is the SINGLE *best interpretation*?

A. Normal
B. Uncompensated metabolic acidosis
C. Partially compensated metabolic acidosis
D. Uncompensated respiratory acidosis
E. Partially compensated respiratory acidosis

320. In one trial, 20/200 people quit smoking with NRT and 10/200 people quit smoking without intervention. What is the absolute risk reduction?

What is the SINGLE *best answer*?

A. 2
B. 5%
C. 10%
D. 20%
E. 50%

321. In another trial, 100/1000 female smokers develop lung cancer. 20/1000 female non-smokers develop lung cancer. What is the absolute risk (incidence) in the general population?

What is the SINGLE *best answer*?

A. 2%
B. 8%
C. 12%
D. 20%
E. 80%

322. What is the relative risk of lung cancer in smokers for Question 321?

What is the SINGLE *best answer*?

A. 0.5
B. 1.5
C. 2
D. 5
E. 8

323. What is the attributable risk of lung cancer for Question 321?

What is the SINGLE *best answer*?

A. 0.08
B. 0.5
C. 0.8
D. 5
E. 8

324. A mother is concerned, as she has read about cot death and SIDS.

What is the SINGLE best *advice you can give her according to the Department of Health*?

A. Lie the baby on his side in the cot
B. Lie the baby in a prone position in the cot with the head at the top of the cot
C. Lie the baby in the supine position in the cot with his feet touching the bottom of the cot
D. Use a sheet alone if the room temperature Is 20°C with a baby in a nappy, vest and babygro
E. Use a sheet + I layer of blankets if the room temperature is 18°C with a baby in a nappy, vest and babygro

325. A 40-year-old woman being treated for rheumatoid arthritis has regular full blood count tests. The latest shows a Hb of 9 g/dl with a mean cell volume of 110 fl.

What is the SINGLE most *likely diagnosis*?

A. Alcoholism
B. Coeliac disease
C. Folate deficiency
D. Pernicious anaemia
E. Vitamin B_{12} deficiency

326. A 30-year-old man complains of being TATT (tired all the time). He is a vegan. FBC shows Hb of 8.5 g/dl with a MCV of 108 fl. Peripheral blood film shows some hypersegmented nuclein in the neutrophils.

What is the SINGLE most *likely diagnosis*?

A. Alcoholism
B. Coeliac disease
C. Folate deficiency
D. Pernicious anaemia
E. Vitamin B$_{12}$ deficiency

327. A mother of a child with sickle cell anaemia asks you what her risk is of having another affected child.

What is the SINGLE *best answer*?

A. 1:1
B. 1:2
C. 1:4
D. 1:8
E. Nil

328. A 9-year-old girl develops *Haemophilus influenzae* type B meningitis.

What is the SINGLE *best advice*?

A. Treat girl alone with benzylpenicillin
B. Treat girl alone with cefotaxime
C. Treat girl and offer prophylactic antibiotics to household members
D. Treat girl and vaccinate all household members
E. Treat girl and vaccinate all household members and school contacts

329. A 30-year-old alcoholic male is brought to Casualty for injuries sustained in a brawl.

What is the SINGLE most *likely radiographic appearance*?

A. Fracture of the distal radius
B. Fractures of the neck of the 4th and 5th metacarpal bones
C. Fracture of the ulna
D. Scaphoid fracture
E. Shoulder dislocation

330. A 30-year-old mother of 3 small children under 5 complains of pain in her right wrist. Pain is elicited with the Finkelstein test.

What is the SINGLE most *likely diagnosis*?

A. Carpal tunnel syndrome
B. DeQuervain's tenosynovitis
C. Dupuytren's contracture
D. Ganglion cyst
E. Trigger thumb

331. A baby is brought to Casualty for fracture of the forearm after allegedly falling from the sofa onto the carpeted floor. The casualty officer suspects NAI. The baby is noted to have blue sclerae. The mother reports that this runs in the family.

What is the SINGLE most *useful investigation*?

A. Genetic testing to locate the mutator gene
B. Refer to ENT for hearing test
C. Skeletal survey
D. Skin biopsy to determine both the quantity and quality of Type I collagen
E. X-ray to confirm spiral fracture

332. A 10-year-old boy complains of eye pain and high fever. On examination, there is periorbital cellulitis and oedema. He explains he had sinus pains 1 week prior.

What is the next most *appropriate investigation*?

A. CT scan
B. Intraocular pressure reading
C. Ishihara colour vision test
D. MRI scan
E. X-ray

333. A 65-year-old woman with chronic atrial fibrillation now presents with a BP of 80/40 and crushing chest pain.

What is the SINGLE most *appropriate management*?

A. Amiodarone
B. Beta-blocker
C. Dofetilide
D. Electrocardioversion
E. Flecainamide

334. A 20-year-old man involved in an RTA on the motorway is brought into Casualty unconscious. BP is 80/50, P 120. CXR shows a widened mediastinum.

What is the SINGLE most *likely diagnosis*?

A. Haemothorax
B. Perforated peptic ulcer
C. Pericardial effusion
D. Ruptured aorta
E. Splenic rupture

335. A man aged 50 and a heavy smoker presents with painless haematuria.

What is the SINGLE *investigation of choice*?

A. DMSA scintigraphy
B. Flexible cystoscopy
C. IV urogram
D. Spiral CT scan
E. Ultrasound

336. A 40-year-old indigent male presents with cough worse in the morning tinged with blood, weight loss and night sweats. CXR shows lower lobe cavitation.

What is the SINGLE most *likely diagnosis*?

A. Bronchiectasis
B. Sarcoidosis
C. Staphylococcal pneumonia
D. Streptococcal pneumonia
E. Tuberculosis

337. A 30-year-old man presents with cough and weight loss. CXR shows perihilar lymph nodes, paratracheal lymph nodes, thickened fissures and decreased lung volumes.

What is the SINGLE most *likely diagnosis*?

A. Hypersensitivity lung disease
B. Lung cancer
C. Sarcoidosis
D. Pneumoconiosis
E. Tuberculosis

338. A 5-year-old girl presents with fever, nosebleeds, and generalised joint pains. On examination, the lymph nodes, liver
and spleen are enlarged.

What is the SINGLE most *likely diagnosis*?

A. Acute lymphocytic leukaemia
B. Acute myeloid leukaemia
C. Chronic lymphocytic leukaemia
D. Chronic myeloid leukaemia
E. Hodgkin's lymphoma

339. A 40-year-old woman with a child with cystic fibrosis would
like antenatal testing to ensure her second child is not
affected.

What is the SINGLE next most *appropriate investigation*?

A. Amniocentesis at 15/40
B. Chorionic villus sampling at 9/40
C. Couples' genetic screening
D. Preimplantation diagnosis
E. Ultrasound

340. A 25-year-old man presents with a non-tender groin lump.
On examination, the lump disappears when the man is lying
supine and re-expands upon standing.

What is the SINGLE most *likely diagnosis*?

A. Epididymal cyst
B. Hernia
C. Hydrocoele
D. Spermatocoele
E. Varicocoele

341. A 20-year-old man reports a thick yellow urethral discharge.
He reports UPSI 3 days ago. He would like empirical treatment before the Gram stain results.

What is the SINGLE most *appropriate treatment*?

A. Acyclovir
B. Ciprofloxacin
C. Doxycycline
D. Metronidazole
E. Penicillin

342. A 55-year-old NIDDM male on metformin is scheduled next morning for pelvic exenteration for extensive rectal carcinoma.

What is the SINGLE most *appropriate pre-operative management of his diabetes?*

A. Increase the dose of metformin
B. Omit morning dose of metformin
C. Start on sliding scale IV insulin
D. Switch to gliclazide MR preparation
E. Switch to SC insulin with hourly fingersticks

343. A 10-year-old girl complains of fever and pains in her wrists and knees. On examination, the cervical lymph nodes and spleen are enlarged.

What is the SINGLE investigation most *likely to be abnormal?*

A. ASO (anti-streptolysin) titres
B. Autoantibodies
C. Bone marrow
D. ESR
E. Philadelphia chromosome

344. A 55-year-old woman complains of inability to close her left eyelid. She is also noted to have vesicles in her left external auditory canal.

What is the SINGLE most *likely affected nerve?*

A. CN II
B. CN III
C. CN IV
D. CN VI
E. CN VII

345. A 50-year-old chronic alcoholic presents with fever and cough. He lives in a homeless shelter. He smokes 20 cigarettes a day and uses an atrovent inhaler.

What is the SINGLE most *appropriate treatment?*

A. Amoxicillin
B. Ciprofloxacin
C. Clarithromycin
D. Doxycycline
E. Prednisolone

346. A woman has a maternal serum screen: AFP, hCG, oestriol and inhibin A. Only the alpha-fetoprotein level comes back high.

What is the SINGLE most *likely potential diagnosis?*

A. Down's syndrome
B. Hydatidiform mole
C. Neural tube defect
D. Normal pregnancy
E. Trisomy 18

347. A 40-year-old woman has an antenatal serum triple marker test. The AFP and oestriol levels are low but the hCG is twice normal.

What is the SINGLE most *likely potential diagnosis?*

A. Down's syndrome
B. Hydatiform mole
C. Neural tube defect
D. Normal pregnancy
E. Trisomy 18

348. A pregnant woman is known to be a hepatitis B carrier.

What is the SINGLE best *management of her baby?*

A. Administer course of hepatitis B vaccination at birth, 1 month and 6 months
B. Administer hepatitis B immunoglobulin and 3-dose course of hepatitis B at birth
C. Administer only hepatitis B immunoglobulin at birth
D. Deliver baby by Caesarian to avoid perinatal transmission of virus
E. Give mother lamivudine in the latter half of pregnancy to prevent perinatal transmission

349. A 55-year-old man presents with breathlessness. You suspect heart failure.

Which SINGLE investigation for heart failure has *been shown to be the most cost effective?*

A. CXR
B. B-type natriuretic peptide
C. Echocardiogram
D. ECG
E. Troponin T

350. A 65-year-old man complains of persistent rectal bleeding.

What is the SINGLE most *appropriate screening test*?

A. Double-contrast barium enema
B. Faecal occult blood
C. Flexible sigmoidoscopy
D. Optical colonoscopy
E. Virtual colonoscopy

351. A 60-year-old man has undergone hemicolectomy for colorectal carcinoma.

What is the SINGLE most *appropriate investigation for cancer surveillance*?

A. 3-monthly CEA tumour marker
B. CT scan
C. Optical colonoscopy
D. PET scan
E. Virtual colonoscopy

352. A 20-year-old man complains of lower back pain of 3 months' duration. On examination, he has pain on SLR at 20 degrees.

What is the SINGLE most *likely diagnosis*?

A. Acute disc disease
B. Inflammatory arthritis
C. Mechanical back pain
D. Non-organic cause
E. Sciatica

353. A 55-year-old obese woman complains of low back pain, which has kept her off work for 4 months. MRI shows L5/S1 mild degenerative disc disease. She has tried NSAIDs, muscle relaxants, diet and physiotherapy to no avail and has even put on weight. There is no radiculopathy.

What is the SINGLE next most *appropriate management*?

A. Lumbar decompression
B. Steroid injections
C. Tramadol
D. Tricyclic antidepressants
E. Vertebroplasty

354. A 70-year-old man with multiple myeloma complains of severe lower back pain. MRI shows pathological fracture lines in 2 lumbar vertebrae.

What is the SINGLE most *appropriate management*?

A. Disc replacement
B. Dynamic stabilisation
C. Lumbar decompression
D. Spinal stabilisation training
E. Vertebroplasty

355. A 30-year-old woman who had an episode of acute otitis media now presents with fever, acute back pain and leg radiculopathy.

What is the SINGLE most *likely diagnosis*?

A. Brucellosis
B. Epidural abscess
C. Pyogenic spondylitis
D. Staphylococcal discitis
E. Tuberculosis

356. A 40-year-old man complains of back pain radiating to his buttocks, worse during the day and aggravated by coughing, sitting or stooping. On examination, there are no radicular symptoms or signs.

What is the SINGLE most *likely diagnosis*?

A. Degenerative spondylolisthesis
B. Discogenic back pain
C. Facet joint arthropathy
D. Mechanical back pain
E. Spinal stenosis

357. A 70-year-old woman complains of back and leg pain when walking. She reports paresthesiae in her leg and weakness. She reports that when she stops walking and rests, the pain is relieved. On examination, the ankle reflexes are absent.

What is the SINGLE most *likely diagnosis*?

A. Degenerative spondylolisthesis
B. Discogenic back pain
C. Facet joint arthropathy
D. Intermittent claudication
E. Spinal stenosis

358. A 50-year-old man complains of morning stiffness. He describes back pain radiating down his buttock and back of thighs. The pain improves with mobilisation. On examination, there is paralumbar tenderness, and the pain is worse on extenstion.

What is the SINGLE most *likely diagnosis*?

A. Ankylosing spondylitis
B. Discogenic back pain
C. Facet joint arthropathy
D. Intermittent claudication
E. Spinal stenosis

359. A 4-year-old girl presents to A&E in distress, with T 40°C. She is sitting forward, unable to speak or swallow, is drooling saliva and turning blue.

What is the SINGLE most *appropriate management*?

A. Administer IM adrenaline 1:1000
B. Administer IV benzylpenicillin
C. Administer IV hydrocortisone
D. Give oxygen and nebulised salbutamol
E. Urgently contact the anaesthetist to intubate the child ASAP

360. A 25-year-old woman requests a UPT for missed period. The test is positive.

What is the SINGLE most *appropriate prescription*?

A. Calcichew forte
B. Ferrous sulphate 200 mg tds
C. Folic acid 400 mcg od
D. Folic acid 5 mg od
E. MVI

361. A 55-year-old woman post vaginal hysterectomy complains of constant urine dribbling.

What is the SINGLE most likely diagnosis?

A. Bladder outlet obstruction
B. Detrusor failure
C. Stress incontinence
D. Uterine prolapse
E. Uterovaginal fistula

362. A 30-year-old woman complains of dribbling urine when she coughs or laughs. She has 3 children under the age of 5.

What is the SINGLE most *appropriate treatment*?

A. Alpha-adrenoreceptor blocker
B. Anticholinergic drug
C. Pelvic floor exercises
D. Ring pessary
E. Topical oestrogen

363. An electrician with a past history of seizures states that he was shocked by a fuse and now presents with shoulder pain.

What is the SINGLE most *likely radiographic appearance*?

A. Anterior shoulder dislocation
B. Fracture of the clavicle
C. Posterior shoulder dislocation
D. Supracondylar fracture of the humerus
E. Surgical neck of humerus fracture

364. A 35-year-old man complains of blood in his stool. There is no family history of CA. There has been no recent travel. He eats a low-residue diet high in protein. On PR exam and proctoscopy, no rectal mass is felt or seen and no haemorrhoids are present. He returns 6 weeks later and reports that the symptoms still persist.

What is the SINGLE most *appropriate management*?

A. Arrange psychiatric consult
B. Check FBC and ESR
C. Reassure him, as he is too young to be at risk of colorectal carcinoma
D. Refer routinely to colorectal clinic for colonoscopy
E. Refer urgently to colorectal clinic for flexible sigmoidoscopy

365. A 30-year-old woman has had 2 consecutive second-trimester miscarriages.

What is the SINGLE most *likely diagnosis*?

A. Antiphospholid antibody positive
B. *Chlamydia* infection
C. Fibroid uterus
D. Incompetent cervix
E. Rhesus incompatibility

366. A 40-year-old woman is brought to A&E with shock and profuse vaginal bleeding. She had delivered her third baby at home. On examination, a low transverse scar is noted.

What is the SINGLE most *likely diagnosis*?

A. Fibroid uterus
B. Postpartum haemorrhage
C. Rhesus incompatibility
D. Ruptured ectopic pregnancy
E. Uterine rupture

367. A 50-year-old woman with metastatic breast cancer complains of severe bone pain. X-ray shows lytic lesions.

What is the SINGLE most *useful modality of pain relief for this patient*?

A. NSAIDs
B. Opioids
C. Radiotherapy
D. Steroid injections
E. TENS

368. A 40-year-old factory worker complains of finger pain. She states she does repetitive motions with her fingers at work and felt her finger click. She reports that now she cannot straighten her finger.

What is the SINGLE most *likely diagnosis*?

A. Boutonniere's deformity
B. Dupuytren's contracture
C. Mallet finger
D. Tendon rupture
E. Trigger finger

369. A 20-year-old netball player complains of pain in her middle finger. She states the ball hit the tip of her finger and bent it backwards. She now cannot straighten the tip of her finger.

What is the SINGLE most *likely diagnosis*?

A. Boutonniere's deformity
B. Dupuytren's contracture
C. Mallet finger
D. Tendon rupture
E. Trigger finger

370. A 30-year-old man presents with a scaly rash on the back of his elbows. He states that the sun seems to improve the rash and when he is stressed the rash is worse.

     What is the SINGLE most *likely diagnosis*?

     A. Discoid eczema
     B. Pityriasis rosacea
     C. Pityriasis versicolor
     D. Psoriasis
     E. Tinea corporis

371. A 55-year-old man was recently started on an anti-hypertensive. He states that now his right big toe is swollen and red. He states arthritis runs in the family.

     What is the SINGLE most *likely culprit*?

     A. Amlodipine
     B. Atenolol
     C. Bendrofluazide
     D. Losartan
     E. Perindopril

372. A 35-year-old mother of two with panic attacks is non-responsive to paroxetine. You decide to try a trial of benzo-diazepine.

     What is the SINGLE most important *side effect you should warn her about*?

     A. Chest pain
     B. Drowsiness the next day
     C. Hallucinations
     D. Night terrors
     E. Photosensitivity

373. A 2-week-old baby is noted to have breast milk jaundice. BR is 16.1 mg/dl indirect and 0.4 mg/dl direct.

     What is the SINGLE most *appropriate management*?

     A. Arrange exchange transfusion
     B. Commence phototherapy
     C. Increase breastfeeding and recheck BR
     D. Stop nursing for 48 hours
     E. Switch to SMA Gold

374. A 20-year-old man returned from holiday and complains of right ear pain. He reports that he swam in the sea. On examination, he has a purulent green otorrhoea. You give him treatment, and he returns the next day complaining of a rash, which developed while he was sunbathing.

What is the SINGLE most *likely diagnosis*?

A. Ciprofloxacin photosensitivity reaction
B. Penicillin allergy
C. Psoriasis
D. Viral rash
E. Weil's disease

375. A 30-year-old man falls off his cycle while racing in a velodrome. He states that it looks like he is looking through murky water. He also notes flashing lights and cannot see down below. He denies pain in his eyes.

What is the SINGLE most *appropriate management*?

A. Administer IV acetazolamide and refer urgently to ophthalmology
B. Apply ocular massage and refer urgently to ophthalmology
C. Refer for laser photocoagulation
D. Tell the patient to lie flat and refer urgently to ophthalmology
E. Treat with steroids

376. A 30-year-old woman's smear test comes back positive for severe dyskaryosis.

What is the SINGLE most *appropriate management*?

A. Refer for colposcopy and biopsy
B. Refer for cone biopsy
C. Refer for LLETZ
D. Repeat smear test in 6 months
E. Repeat smear test in 1 year

377. A 40-year-old woman's smear test comes back positive for CIN II.

What is the SINGLE most *appropriate management*?

A. Refer for colposcopy and biopsy
B. Refer for cone biopsy
C. Refer for LLETZ
D. Repeat smear test in 6 months
E. Repeat smear test in 1 year

378. A 70-year-old female with chronic arthritis is taking arthrotec. She now presents with flank pain, polyuria, nocturia, and cloudy, bloody urine.

What is the SINGLE most *likely diagnosis*?

A. Acute glomerulonephritis
B. Acute pyelonephritis
C. IgA nephropathy
D. Interstitial nephritis
E. Renal papillary necrosis

379. A 65-year-old man complains of low mood for 2 years. He has poor appetite and poor self-esteem. He has difficulty concentrating and is slightly irritable and anxious.

What is the SINGLE most *likely diagnosis*?

A. Alzheimer's disease
B. Dysthymic disorder
C. Frontal dementia
D. Lewy body disorder
E. Pick's disease

380. A 60-year-old alcoholic presents with confusion and ataxia. On examination, the pupils are miotic and non-reactive. There are both vertical and horizontal nystagmus and complete loss of ocular movements.

What is the SINGLE most *appropriate management*?

A. Burr hole
B. CT scan to exclude subdural haematoma
C. Folate
D. IV hydrocortisone
E. Thiamine

381. A 65-year-old heavy smoker reports weight loss (2 stone in 2 months), jaundice, fatigue, and loss of appetite. On examination, there is epigastric tenderness. Investigations reveal low glucose.

What is the SINGLE most *likely diagnosis*?

A. Acute pancreatitis
B. Gastric adenocarcinoma
C. Pancreatic carcinoma
D. Perforated peptic ulcer
E. VIPoma

382. A 50-year-old woman complains of dry, red, itchy eyes and a dry mouth. She describes her mouth as full of cotton. She also has a history of arthritis and muscle pain. Schirmer test shows 5 mm of tears.

What is the SINGLE most *likely diagnosis*?

A. Diabetes
B. Rheumatoid arthritis
C. Sjögren's syndrome
D. SLE
E. Vitamin A deficiency

383. A 40-year-old woman in her second trimester has a scan, which reveals double-bubble sign, shortened humerus and femur, and mild cerebral ventriculomegaly.

What is the SINGLE most *appropriate diagnostic test for this patient at this time*?

A. Amniocentesis
B. Chorionic villus sampling
C. Scan findings conclusive for condition so no diagnostic test required
D. Scan for nuchal fold thickness
E. Triple maternal serum test

384. A 25-year-old woman complains of tremor, palpitations, weight loss, and heat intolerance.

What is the SINGLE most *appropriate investigation*?

A. Chest x-ray
B. 12-lead ECG
C. 24-hour Holter monitoring
D. Thyroid function tests
E. Ultrasound of neck

385. An 80-year-old man complains of breathlessness when he sits up, which is relieved when he is lying down. Pulse ox shows normal O_2 when lying but a sharp reduction upon sitting up.

What is the SINGLE investigation most *likely to provide a definitive diagnosis*?

A. Chest x-ray
B. 12-lead ECG
C. 24-hour Holter monitoring
D. Transthoracic echo
E. V/Q scan

386. A 45-year-old man is undergoing laparascopic live donor nephrectomy. Four endoscopic ports are used: one in the umbilicus, one between the umbilicus and xiphoid process, one in the flank and one midway between the umbilicus and anterior superior iliac spine. The last port traverses which structures?

What is the SINGLE *best answer*?

A. External oblique aponeurosis and internal oblique muscles
B. Linea transversae
C. Poupart's ligament
D. Pyramidalis muscle
E. Transversus abdominus

387. A 46-year-old woman informs you that her mother was diagnosed with ovarian cancer at age 55. She is concerned, as she now smokes, drinks and is on HRT.

What is the SINGLE most *appropriate management*?

A. Advise her to stop drinking as it is a risk factor for ovarian CA
B. Advise her to stop HRT as it doubles the risk of ovarian CA
C. Advise her to stop smoking as it is a risk factor for ovarian CA
D. Refer her for genetic testing
E. Test for CA-125

388. A 55-year-old woman complains of difficulty swallowing, vomiting, weight loss and melena. On examination, there is a supraclavicular lymph node and a hyperpigmented velvety plaque in her axilla.

What is the SINGLE most *likely malignancy*?

A. Gastric carcinoma
B. Laryngeal carcinoma
C. Oesophageal carcinoma
D. Pancreatic carcinoma
E. Thyroid carcinoma

389. An 8-year-old girl presents with several echymoses on her body. The mother and girl deny any trauma. The mother reports that the girl has also had several lengthy episodes of nosebleeds.

What is the SINGLE most *appropriate management*?

A. Chromosome karyotyping
B. Obtain a skeletal survey
C. Refer to child protection services for NAI
D. Take blood for FBC and clotting screen
E. No investigation or treatment required

390. An 18-month-old boy presents with a hoarse barking cough and inspiratory stridor.

What is the SINGLE most *likely organism*?

A. Coxsackievirus
B. *Haemophilus influenzae*
C. Influenza virus type A
D. *Mycoplasma* pneumonia
E. *Parainfluenzavirus*

391. A 40-year-old female takes an overdose of 30 tablets. She complains of nausea and vomiting. 12 hours later she is noted to be jaundiced, confused and lapses into a coma.

What is the SINGLE most *likely poison*?

A. Codeine
B. Coproxamol
C. Ibuprofen
D. Paracetamol
E. Tricyclic antidepressant

392. A 30-year-old woman being treated for bipolar disorder now develops ataxia and elevated hepatic and renal enzymes.

What is the SINGLE most *likely culprit*?

A. Carbamazepine
B. Lithium
C. Olanzapine
D. Risperidone
E. Sodium valproate

393. A heroin misuser presents with fever and nonproductive cough. CXR shows diffuse bilateral interstitial infiltrates.

What is the SINGLE most *appropriate medication*?

A. Amoxicillin
B. Clindamycin
C. Dapsone
D. Prednisolone
E. Trimethoprim-sulfamethoxazole

394. A 40-year-old man presents with lower back pain and no radiculopathy. He is anxious and would like to know what percentage of patients shows a full recovery.

What is the SINGLE best answer?

A. 67%
B. 70%
C. 80%
D. 90%
E. 100%

395. What is the SINGLE most *appropriate management for this man*? (Same patient as question 394)

A. Prescribe benzodiazepine and NSAIDs
B. Refer him to a chiropractor
C. Refer him to physiotherapist
D. Strict bedrest for 2 weeks
E. Take regular paracetamol and keep active

396. A 70-year-old woman is witnessed collapsing. She turned deathly pale before she lost consciousness and fell. The witness rushed to her side and noted a slow pulse.

What is the SINGLE most *likely diagnosis*?

A. Carotid sinus syndrome
B. Epilepsy
C. Hypoglycaemia
D. Stokes-Adams attack
E. Vertebrobasilar ischaemia

397. What is the SINGLE definitive *treatment for this patient*? (Same patient as question 396)

A. Carbamazepine
B. Carotid artery ligation
C. Carotid sinus massage
D. Implantable pacemaker
E. Soft collar

398. A 70-year-old woman with osteoarthritis presents with transient episodes of dizziness and fainting, loss of balance, difficulty walking, nausea and transient global amnesia.

What is the SINGLE most *likely diagnosis*?

A. Carotid sinus syndrome
B. Multi-infarct dementia
C. Pick's disease
D. Stokes-Adams attack
E. Vertebrobasilar ischaemia

399. A 4-year-old girl presents with bloody diarrhoea and seizures. She had been visiting a farm recently. Her BP is raised and she stops making urine. Blood tests reveal anaemia, decreased platelets and haemolytic anaemia Coombs test is negative.

What is the SINGLE most *likely diagnosis*?

A. Haemolytic uraemic syndrome
B. Infectious mononucleosis
C. SLE
D. Thalassaemia
E. Thrombotic thrombocytopenic purpura

400. A 40-year-old woman presents with a photosensitive rash, joint pain and painless nose ulcers. Tests reveal proteinuria with casts in the urine.

What is the SINGLE investigation most *likely to provide a definitive diagnosis*?

A. Anti-mitochondrial antibody
B. Anti-nuclear antibody
C. Endomysial antibodies
D. ESR
E. Rheumatoid factor

401. While on paediatric ward rounds, you see a 7-year-old girl start turning blue. She is grabbing her throat. There is a breakfast tray at her bedside.

What is the SINGLE most *appropriate management*?

A. Administer adrenaline 1:1000 IM
B. Administer the Heimlich manouevre
C. Bleep the anaesthetist to intubate her
D. Bleep ENT to perform a tracheostomy
E. Place the girl over your lap and slap her back

402. A 30-year-old seatbelted passenger involved in a high-speed RTA comes in with abdominal pain and bruising over the 11th and 12th ribs on her left side.

What is the SINGLE most *appropriate management*?

A. Arrange for urgent laparotomy
B. Arrange urgent IVP
C. Obtain abdominal CT scan
D. Obtain abdominal ultrasound
E. Obtain upright CXR

403. A 35-year-old seat-belted driver involved in a high speed RTA complains of chest pains. On examination, there is bruising over the chest along the lines of the seat belt. Troponin and CK-MB enzymes return elevated and ECG shows first-degree heartblock.

What is the SINGLE next most *appropriate investigation*?

A. Aortogram
B. Chest CT scan
C. Thoracic ultrasound
D. Transoesophageal echocardiogram
E. Transthoracic echocardiogram

404. A 2-year-old child is brought into Casualty after swallowing a 50p coin. X-ray confirms the presence of an opaque object at the cricopharyngeal sphincter. There are no respiratory symptoms.

What is the SINGLE next most *appropriate management*?

A. Encourage child to drink fizzy drinks and give buscopan IM
B. Reassure mother that coin will eventually pass
C. Refer to ENT to remove under GA
D. Refer to GI to remove with endoscopy
E. Remove using laryngoscope

405. A 40-year-old woman complains of fishy-smelling offensive vaginal discharge. Microscopy shows the presence of clue cells.

What is the SINGLE most *appropriate treatment*?

A. Advise to stop bubble-baths and douching and it will clear spontaneously
B. Prescribe clotrimazole pessary and cream
C. Prescribe ciprofloxacin
D. Prescribe doxycycline
E. Prescribe metronidazole

406. A 40-year-old man complains of fever, confusion and dysphagia since returning from Mexico. CXR reveals a widened mediastinum with air–fluid level behind an enlarged heart. Barium swallow shows a tortuous widened food-filled oesophagus.

What is the SINGLE most *likely diagnosis*?

A. Achalasia
B. Oesophageal varices
C. Perforated peptic ulcer
D. Ruptured aorta
E. *Trypanosoma cruzi* (Chagas' disease)

407. A 35-year-old firefighter suffering from 30% burns, complains of epigastric pain. Endoscopy reveals multiple small superficial ulcers.

What is the SINGLE most *likely diagnosis*?

A. Atrophic gastritis
B. Barrett's metaplasia
C. Curling's ulcer
D. Cushing's ulcer
E. Perforated peptic ulcer

408. A 70-year-old man returns from holiday in the US and has vague chest pain and mild breathlessness. On examination, JVP is raised. BP is 110/60, P 120. ECG shows Q-wave and T-wave inversion in lead 3.

What is the SINGLE most *likely diagnosis*?

A. Acute MI
B. Acute pericarditis
C. Acute pulmonary embolism
D. Cardiac tamponade
E. Pulmonary contusion

409. A 55-year-old man complains that he can't breathe at night. JVP is raised. On examination, basal creps are auscultated. CXR shows blunting of the costophrenic angles and small effusion.

What is the SINGLE most *likely diagnosis*?

A. Basilar pneumonia
B. Haemothorax
C. Pulmonary contusion
D. Pulmonary embolism
E. Pulmonary oedema

410. A 12-year-old Indian girl presents with a neck lump. FNAC reveals caseating granuloma.

What is the SINGLE most *appropriate treatment*?

A. Chemotherapy
B. Isoniazid, rifampicin and pyrazidamide
C. Prednisolone
D. Terbinafine
E. Vaccination against tuberculosis

411. A 70-year-old man is noted to have a serum potassium level of 7.5 mmol/l and is unable to pass urine. On examination the bladder is not palpable. Urea and creatinine levels are also extremely high. ECG shows progressive bradycardia and peak Ts.

What is the SINGLE most *appropriate treatment*?

A. Cation-exchange resin
B. Dialysis
C. IV calcium
D. IV glucose and insulin
E. Sodium bicarbonate

412. A 20-year-old woman complains of frequent episodes of palpitations and dizziness. She comes into A&E as the current episode persists. On examination the pulse rate is 180. ECG confirms SVT. She has a history of asthma.

What is the SINGLE most *useful treatment*?

A. Adenosine
B. Beta-blocker
C. Catheter ablation treatment
D. Digoxin
E. Verapamil

413. A 30-year-old man is struck in his temple by a cricket ball and suffers a fractured skull. He is initially lucid but then loses consciousness.

What is the SINGLE *artery that is most at risk*?

A. Anterior cerebral artery
B. Internal carotid artery
C. Middle cerebral artery
D. Middle meningeal artery
E. Superficial temporal artery

414. A 70-year-old frail woman has incidental findings of bruising on both her wrists and upper back. She denies trauma and is timid. She lives with her son's family.

What is the SINGLE most *likely cause*?

A. Bleeding disorder
B. Cirrhosis
C. Elder abuse
D. Leukemia
E. Scurvy

415. An 18-month-old boy had a single MMR jab 1 week ago and now presents with fever, non-blanching rash and drowsiness.

What is the SINGLE most *likely cause*?

A. Henoch-Schönlein purpura
B. Kawasaki's disease
C. Meningitis
D. Reaction to vaccine
E. Toxic shock syndrome

416. A 4-year-old Korean girl presents with 5 days of fever. T = 40°C. There is a swollen purple-red rash on her palms and soles and swollen tongue with sores in her mouth. The mother reports that she has noticed the skin start to peel on the palms.

What is the SINGLE most *likely diagnosis*?

A. Henoch-Schönlein purpura
B. Kawasaki's disease
C. Meningitis
D. Staphylococcal scalded skin syndrome
E. Toxic shock syndrome

417. A 20-year-old driver involved in a high-speed RTA presents with facial nerve palsy, conductive hearing loss and clear discharge from his right ear.

What is the SINGLE most *likely diagnosis*?

A. Basilar skull fracture
B. Extradural haematoma
C. Longitudinal temporal bone fracture
D. Subdural haematoma
E. Transverse temporal bone fracture

418. A 10-year-old boy is accidentally struck in the head by a cricket bat and now presents to Casualty with raccoon/panda eyes (bruising around the eyes), Battle's sign (bruising behind the ear tracking down the neck) and blood behind the tympanic membrane. He has clear discharge coming from his nose.

What is the SINGLE most *likely diagnosis*?

A. Basilar skull fracture
B. Extradural haematoma
C. Longitudinal temporal bone fracture
D. Subdural haematoma
E. Transverse temporal bone fracture

419. A 45-year-old woman reports nipple changes. On examination, there are scaly, erythematous plaques on and around the inverted nipple. On squeezing the nipple, a serosanguinous discharge appears.

What is the SINGLE most *likely diagnosis*?

A. Amyloidosis
B. Contact dermatitis
C. Eczema
D. Mastitis
E. Paget's disease

420. A 35-year-old multip. 27/40 presents with painless bright red PVB and hypotension.

What is the SINGLE most *likely diagnosis*?

A. Abruptio placenta
B. DIC
C. Inevitable miscarriage
D. Placenta praevia
E. Uterine rupture

421. A 55-year-old woman complains of blurry vision. Fundoscopic exam reveals macular pigmentation. + Amsler grid test distortion. Fluorescein angiogram confirms the diagnosis.

What is the SINGLE most *useful treatment*?

A. Laser photocoagulation
B. Oral steroids
C. Photodynamic therapy
D. Radiation therapy
E. Transpupillary thermotherapy

422. A 35-year-old woman with lupus now reports that she has blurry vision and photophobia. On examination, the orbit is tender to palpation. The engorged blood vessels do not blanch with phenylephrine.

What is the SINGLE most *likely diagnosis*?

A. Episcleritis
B. Keratitis
C. Keratoconjunctivitis sicca
D. Scleritis
E. Uveitis

423. A 40-year-old mother of 3 would like the Mirena IUS for contraception. She would like to know its mode of action.

What is the SINGLE *best answer*?

A. Alteration of cervical mucus
B. Inhibition of implantation of an egg and thickening of cervical mucus
C. Inhibition of ovulation
D. Inhibition of ovulation and implantation
E. Spermicidal

424. A 25-year-old woman would like to know the mode of action of the mini-pill.

What is the SINGLE *best answer*?

A. Alteration of cervical mucus
B. Inhibition of implantation of an egg and thickening of cervical mucus
C. Inhibition of ovulation
D. Inhibition of ovulation and implantation
E. Spermicidal

425. A 50-year-old man complains of loss of taste. On examination, there is loss of taste of the anterior two-thirds of the tongue and loss of secretion of submandibular and sublingual glands.

What is the SINGLE most *likely diagnosis*?

A. Bell's palsy
B. Lesion of chorda tympani
C. Lesion of lingual nerve
D. Lesion of CN VII at the internal acoustic meatus
E. Lesion of CN VII at the stylomastoid foramen

426. A 6-year-old girl sustains a midshaft fracture of the humerus and presents with a wrist drop.

What is the SINGLE most *likely diagnosis*?

A. Axillary nerve palsy
B. Median nerve palsy
C. Musculocutaneous nerve palsy
D. Radial nerve palsy
E. Ulnar nerve palsy

427. A 35-year-old female with SLE presents with high BP and renal failure. Histology shows proliferation of endothelial cells, leukocyte infiltration and crescent-shaped cells extending out of Bowman's capsule.

What is the SINGLE most *likely diagnosis*?

A. Amyloidosis
B. Haemolytic uraemic syndrome
C. IgA nephropathy
D. Nephrotic syndrome
E. Rapidly progressive glomerulonephritis

428. A 2-year-old boy presents with painless jelly-like blood in his stool. FBC shows an iron-deficiency anaemia.

What is the SINGLE most *likely diagnosis*?

A. Angiodysplasia
B. Intussusception
C. Meckel's diverticulum
D. Pyloric stenosis
E. Ulcerative colitis

429. A 55-year-old man 1 week post CABG presents with sharp central chest pain. The pain is relieved by leaning forward or standing with a straight back. It is worse when breathing in or lying back. ECG shows diffuse concave upward ST segment changes.

What is the SINGLE most *likely diagnosis*?

A. Acute pulmonary embolism
B. Cardiac tamponade
C. Costochondritis
D. Dressler's syndrome
E. Ventricular rupture

430. A 55-year-old heavy smoker needs to be assessed prior to cholecystectomy. He uses an ipratropium inhaler. Vital signs are stable. CXR is normal.

What is the SINGLE most *important pre-operative investigation*?

A. Arterial blood gas
B. Lung function tests (spirometry)
C. Peak flow rate
D. Pulse oximetry
E. CT scan chest

431. A 60-year-old man complains of lower back pain radiating down his left leg. On exam, there is an absent ankle jerk and loss of sensation over the lateral border and the sole of the foot.

What is the SINGLE most *likely affected nerve or nerve root*?

A. L3
B. L4
C. L5
D. S1
E. Lateral femoral cutaneous nerve

432. A 40-year-old woman on risperidone complains of galactorrhoea, absence of periods, decreased libido and inability to conceive for the past year.

What is the SINGLE most *useful investigation*?

A. CT scan of the head
B. MRI of pituitary
C. Prolactin levels
D. Thyroid function tests
E. Transvaginal ultrasound

433. A 40-year-old woman complains of frontal headache, muscle weakness and polyuria. On exam, BP is 180/100. Muscle power is reduced. Routine blood tests reveal a low potassium and metabolic acidosis. The aldosterone is high, and the plasma renin is low.

What is the SINGLE most *likely diagnosis*?

A. Cushing's disease
B. Conn's syndrome
C. Parathyroid adenoma
D. Phaeochromocytoma
E. Renal artery stenosis

434. A 40-year-old man from India complains of blurry vision and eye pain. On examination, there is blepharospasm, photophobia, and excessive tearing. You diagnosis interstitial keratitis.

What is the SINGLE most *appropriate treatment*?

A. Acyclovir
B. Sodium stiboglutinate
C. Penicillin
D. Topical antibiotic drops
E. Topical corticosteroid drops

435. A 30-year-old woman who wears contact lenses now complains of eye pain. Fluorescein dye shows uptake.

What is the SINGLE most *useful treatment*?

A. Topical anaesthetic
B. Topical analgaesic
C. Topical corticosteroids
D. Topical gentamicin
E. Topical neomycin

436. A 6-month-old baby presents with a high fever. On examination, T = 40°C with no obvious nidus of infection. She is agitated and inconsolable. She is not her usual self, according to the mother, and has been off her food. The temperature remains high in Casualty despite administration of Calpol.

What is the SINGLE most *appropriate management*?

A. Admit for full work-up – blood cultures, routine bloods, CXR and UA
B. Give baby Nurofen and keep in A&E for further observation
C. Reassure mother that it is viral and send baby home with Nurofen
D. Send baby home with amoxicillin
E. Send baby home with Calpol, and request mother bring back baby's urine sample

437. This condition has an incidence of 15% in females over the age of 50, 30% in females over the age of 70 and 40% in females over the age of 80.

What is the SINGLE most *likely condition*?

A. Back pain
B. Breast cancer
C. COPD
D. Lung cancer
E. Osteoporosis

438. What is the SINGLE *leading cause of mortality among women in the UK*?

A. Breast cancer
B. Circulatory diseases
C. Infectious diseases
D. Lung cancer
E. Respiratory diseases

439. A 35-year-old multip. has postpartum haemorrhage of 550 ml following removal of the placenta.

What is the SINGLE most *appropriate management*?

A. Administer 10 IU syntocinon IM
B. Administer 10 IU syntocinon IV bolus
C. Commence 40 IU syntocinon IV drip diluted in 500 ml Hartmann's solution at 125 ml/h
D. Take to theatre for EUA
E. Transfuse blood

440. A 25-year-old primip. fails to progress in the first stage of labour.

What is the SINGLE most *appropriate management*?

A. Administer 10 IU syntocinon IM
B. Administer 10 IU syntocinon IV bolus
C. Administer 10 IU syntocinon in 500 ml Hartmann's at 6 ml/h and increase by 6 ml every 15 minutes
D. Administer 10 IU syntocinon in 500 ml Hartmann's at 6 ml/h and increase by 6 ml every 30 minutes
E. Take to theatre for Caesarian section

441. According to BMJ Clinical Evidence, the incidence of this disease is > 70% and is most common between the ages of 35 and 55. 70% will return to work within 1 week and 90% within 2 months.

What is the SINGLE most *likely condition with this profile*?

A. Depression
B. Influenza
C. Mechanical back pain
D. Repetitive strain injury
E. Stress

442. A 20-year-old nullip. woman presents with deep dyspareunia for months. She reports that her cycles are short but last for 8 days. She has pain a few days before her period is due and for 2 days into the period. On examination, there is adnexal tenderness but no cervical motion excitation. She is married. She is a nonsmoker.

What is the SINGLE most *useful investigation*?

A. Endocervical swab
B. High vaginal swab
C. Laparoscopy
D. Pap smear
E. Transvaginal ultrasound

443. A 35-year-old woman with a history of endometriosis now presents with severe right-sided lower abdominal pain and nausea. T = 37°C, BP 80/50, P 130. On examination, the abdomen is distended with rebound tenderness and guarding, and appears gravid. On internal examination, there is right adnexal tenderness and fullness. UPT is negative. There is no PVB.

What is the SINGLE most *likely diagnosis*?

A. Hydatidiform mole
B. Red degeneration of fibroid
C. Ruptured appendicitis
D. Ruptured ectopic pregnancy
E. Ruptured ovarian cyst

444. A 14-year-old boy has signs of mental retardation. On examination, he has a prominent forehead, ears and chin. He is also noted to have a mid-systolic heart murmur and large testes. DNA analysis reveals > 200 trinucleotide repeat expansion of one particular gene.

What is the SINGLE most *likely diagnosis*?

A. Autism
B. Down's syndrome
C. Fragile X syndrome
D. Prader-Willi syndrome
E. Tuberous sclerosis

445. A 14-year-old boy falls from a tree onto a dorsiflexed wrist. He complains of wrist pain. PA and lateral X-rays confirm perilunate dislocation.

What is the SINGLE most *appropriate treatment*?

A. Closed reduction and casting
B. Closed reduction and percutaneous pin fixation
C. Open reduction and ligamentous repair with percutaneous pin fixation
D. Plaster cast for 6 weeks
E. Strapping for 2 weeks

446. A 30-year-old heroin misuser presents with fever, drowsiness and neck stiffness. On examination, a heart murmur is noted and Janeway lesions on the palms (red, painless spots). Brudzinski (forced neck flexion leads to flexion at the hip and knee) and Kernig signs (inability to extend legs) are present. CSF from a lumbar puncture reveals leukocytosis with neutrophils, high protein and low glucose.

What is the SINGLE most *likely diagnosis*?

A. Meningococcal meningitis
B. Staphylococcal meningitis
C. Subacute bacterial endocarditis
D. Tuberculosis
E. Viral meningitis

447. A 7-year-old girl has a distance squint. On examination, the right eye deviates outward when looking at a fixed object in the distance.

What is the SINGLE most *appropriate treatment*?

A. Concave lens for myopia
B. Convex lens for hyperopia
C. Patch left eye
D. Reassure mother that child will grow out of squint.
E. Surgery

448. A 30-year-old woman presents with fever, pain, and an erythematous, discharging wound at the site of an insect bite on her arm. Gram stain reveals Gram-positive non-motile organism in chains.

What is the SINGLE most *likely organism*?

A. *Bacillus anthracis*
B. *Staphylococcus aureus*
C. *Staphylococcus epidermidis*
D. *Streptococcus pneumoniae*
E. *Streptococcus pyogenes*

449. A 40-year-old man presents with fever, pain, oedema and erythema of his lower leg. On examination, there is purple discolouration of the skin around an insect bite with erythema extending up his leg and a black spot on the leg. The edges are not well demarcated. The skin and subcutaneous tissues start to loosen and a putrid discharge develops. X-ray shows subcutaneous gas.

What is the SINGLE most *likely diagnosis*?

A. Cellulitis
B. Erysipelas
C. Gas gangrene
D. Necrotising fasciitis
E. Toxic shock syndrome

450. A 30-year-old woman complains of fever, dry cough and muscle pains. She states that she attended a work conference at a spa resort in October and has not felt the same since and nor have her female colleagues at the conference. This was 1 week ago.

What is the SINGLE most *likely diagnosis*?

A. *Haemophilus* influenza
B. *Legionella* pneumonia
C. Seasonal influenza
D. Streptococcal pneumonia
E. URTI

451. A 34-year-old pregnant woman would like to be screened for Down's syndrome baby. She says that her older sister has a Down's baby and she is worried.

What is the SINGLE most *appropriate screening test*?

A. Amniocentesis
B. Chorionic villus sampling
C. Nil. Reassure that her risk is insignificant
D. Triple test (bHCG, oestriol and AFP)
E. Ultrasound for nuchal fold thickness

452. A 30-year-old slim woman with 3 children under 5, presents with a painless groin lump. She states that it expands on coughing or straining and that she can push it back in. She reports a dragging sensation. The lump is above and medial to the pubic tubercle. On invagination of the labia, the lump is palpated on the tip of the examining finger.

What is the SINGLE most *likely diagnosis*?

A. Bartholin's cyst
B. Direct inguinal hernia
C. Femoral hernia
D. Indirect inguinal hernia
E. Saphena varix

453. A 6-week-old baby boy presents with frequent projectile non-bilious vomiting.

What is the SINGLE most *likely acid-base disturbance in this baby*?

A. Metabolic acidosis
B. Metabolic alkalosis
C. Respiratory acidosis
D. Respiratory alkalosis
E. Mixed metabolic and respiratory disturbance

454. What is the SINGLE *investigation of choice for suspected pyloric stenosis*?

A. Barium enema
B. CT scan of the abdomen
C. Endoscopy
D. Ultrasound
E. Upper GI series

455. A 55-year-old fireman has scratched his hand against a rusty soiled farm ladder and now presents with an open wound 24 hours later. He had tetanus vaccine 10 years ago.

What is the SINGLE most *appropriate management*?

A. Administer human anti-tetanus immunoglobulin, penicillin and metronidazole
B. Administer a single reinforcing dose of tetanus vaccine, penicillin and metronidazole
C. Administer human anti-tetanus immunoglobulin and a single reinforcing dose of tetanus vaccine
D. Administer human anti-tetanus immunoglobulin, penicillin, metronidazole and a single reinforcing dose of tetanus vaccine
E. Administer penicillin and metronidazole alone as patient does not have symptoms of tetanus

456. A 60-year-old man with ischaemic heart disease and emphysema is scheduled for phacoemulsification cataract surgery.

What is the SINGLE most *appropriate form of anaesthesia*?

A. General anaesthesia
B. Epidural anaesthesia
C. Orbital injection
D. Topical anaesthesia
E. Topical anaesthesia and IV sedation

457. A 7-year-old boy presents with a painful limp. On examination, there is limited hip internal rotation and abduction. Rolling the hip into internal rotation elicits pain.

What is the SINGLE most *likely diagnosis*?

A. Legg–Calvé–Perthes disease
B. Metaphyseal dysplasia
C. Septic arthritis
D. Sickle cell anaemia
E. Slipped femoral capital epiphysis

458. A 13-year-old obese boy presents with left hip pain. A week ago the pain started in his left knee.

What is the SINGLE most *likely radiographic finding on lateral frog-leg view*?

A. Juvenile rheumatoid arthritis
B. Legg–Calvé–Perthes disease
C. Nil as this is muscle strain
D. Osgood-Schlatter disease
E. Slipped femoral capital epiphysis

459. A 40-year-old 34/40 woman is noted to have an incidental BP of 160/100 on an antenatal review. She denies blurry vision. There is no proteinuria and no signs of peripheral oedema. Blood tests are normal.

What is the SINGLE most *appropriate management*?

A. Admit to hospital
B. Commence hydralazine
C. Commence labetalol
D. Commence methyldopa
E. Commence nifedipine

460. A 55-year-old woman requests HRT for menopausal symptoms of hot flushes and night sweats. Her last menses was 2 years ago. She would like a non-bleed prep.

What is the SINGLE most *appropriate medication*?

A. Premarin
B. Premique
C. Prempak C
D. Raloxifene
E. Tibolone

461. A 21/40 pregnant female complains of headache, nausea and vomiting. BP is 150/100. On examination, there is right upper quadrant abdominal tenderness. Blood test reveals a platelet count of 80,000, with total BR 1.5 mg/dl, SGOT 80 IU/L and LDH 650 IU/L.

What is the SINGLE most *likely diagnosis*?

A. Eclampsia
B. Fitz-Hugh–Curtis syndrome
C. HELLP syndrome
D. Hepatitis
E. SLE

462. A 17-year-old woman post-delivery requests contraception. She plans to breast-feed.

What is the SINGLE most *appropriate contraceptive advice*?

A. Coc at 3 weeks post delivery
B. Condoms only
C. Depo-provera at 6 weeks
D. Implanon at 6 weeks
E. POP at 3 weeks

463. A 44-year-old man with moderate depression non-responsive to SSRIs is advised by psychiatry to commence venlafaxine. BP is 130/80.

What is the SINGLE *mandatory investigation before commencing this drug*?

A. ABG
B. CXR
C. 12-lead ECG
D. TFT
E. Urea/lytes

464. A 14-year-old girl has a BMI of 14. She has lanugo hair, bradycardia and a distorted self-image; she insists she is still overweight.

What is the SINGLE most *likely acid-base disturbance in this patient*?

A. Hyperchloraemic metabolic acidosis
B. Hyperkalaemic metabolic acidosis
C. Hypochloraemic metabolic alkalosis
D. Hypokalaemic hypochloraemic metabolic alkalosis
E. Respiratory acidosis

465. A 30-year-old woman on lithium is told to get her lithium levels checked. She wants to know how long after she takes the lithium should she have her blood test.

What is the SINGLE *best answer*?

A. 2 hours
B. 4 hours
C. 6 hours
D. 8 hours
E. 12 hours

466. A 50-year-old woman notices slurred speech, a tendency to drop things at work and muscle cramps. On examination, dysarthria, muscle atrophy of the lower limbs, radiculopathy and muscle fasciculations at rest are noted.

What is the SINGLE most *likely diagnosis*?

A. Guillain–Barré syndrome
B. Ischaemic stroke
C. Motor neuron disease
D. Multiple sclerosis
E. Myasthaenia gravis

467. A 30-year-old female presents with SOB. CXR reveals radio-translucency on the right with absence of vascular markings.

What is the SINGLE most *likely diagnosis*?

A. Acute pulmonary embolism
B. Acute pulmonary oedema
C. Haemothorax
D. Pneumonia
E. Pneumothorax

468. A 70-year-old female complains of dysphagia to solids. She states that when her GP started her on iron the dysphagia improved.

What is the SINGLE most *likely diagnosis*?

A. Globus pharyngeus
B. Pharyngeal pouch
C. Plummer-Vinson syndrome/Patterson-Brown Kelly syndrome
D. Post-cricoid carcinoma
E. Zenker diverticulum

469. A 16-year-old boy is punched in the eye and complains of blurry vision.

What is the SINGLE most *likely finding*?

A. Corneal abrasion
B. Hyphaema
C. Retinal detachment
D. Subconjunctival haemorrhage
E. Vitreous haemorrhage

470. An 11-year-old girl falls off her bicycle at high speed, turns pale and has transient loss of vision. The father comes to you as he is concerned and wants to know what happened.

What is the SINGLE most *likely diagnosis*?

A. Hypoglycaemic attack
B. Petit mal seizure
C. Postural syncope
D. Psychogenic syncope
E. Vasovagal attack

471. A 50-year-old alcoholic presents with profuse epistaxis.

What is the SINGLE most *likely blood abnormality*?

A. Abnormal platelet aggregation test
B. Decreased platelets
C. Increased activated partial thromboplastin time
D. Increased bleeding time
E. Increased prothrombin time

472. A 50-year-old woman post THR presents with tachypnoea. PCWP is 22 mmHg. On chest examination, there are bilateral rales. Urine output is 10 ml/hour.

What is the SINGLE most *definitive management*?

A. Administer bendrofluazide p.o.
B. Administer frusemide IV
C. Administer nifedipine p.o.
D. Arrange CXR
E. Do ABG

473. A 60-year-old obese woman post oesophagogastrectomy for oesophageal carcinoma is noted to have a BP of 90/50, P 100 in the recovery room. She is alert postoperatively. She is on a morphine PCA. Urine in the Foley bag is concentrated. The abdomen has no bowel sounds and is distended. Her extremities are cold. FBC is 10 g/dl. She then suddenly loses consciousness.

What is the SINGLE most *likely diagnosis*?

A. Cardiac tamponade
B. DIC
C. Pulmonary embolism
D. Septic shock
E. Splenic artery injury (iatrogenic)

474. A 16-year-old girl presents with haematuria. She reports that she had a bout of tonsillitis 1 week ago. UA also shows proteinuria.

What is the SINGLE most *likely diagnosis?*

A. Alport syndrome
B. IgA nephropathy
C. Lupus nephritis
D. Poststreptococcal glomerulonephritis
E. Rapidly progressive glomerulonephritis

475. A 10-month-old baby is noted to still have a head lag when pulled into a sitting position and cannot sit by himself. He holds his left hand in a clenched fist. Muscle tone is decreased with increased reflexes. He has excessive drooling.

What is the SINGLE most *likely diagnosis?*

A. Cerebral palsy
B. Down's syndrome
C. Duchenne's muscular dystrophy
D. Fragile X syndrome
E. Neurofibromatosis

476. A 100-year-old woman presents with profuse epistaxis. Initial BP is 200/100. After initial resuscitation, BP is brought down to 160/90.

What is the SINGLE next most *appropriate management?*

A. 4 cm Merocel nasal packing (anterior)
B. 8 cm Merocel nasal packing (anterior)
C. Blood transfusion
D. Brighton balloons (posterior tamponade)
E. Foley catheter (posterior tamponade)

477. A 35-year-old woman with toxic multinodular goitre is being prepared for surgery for treatment of thyrotoxicosis.

What is the SINGLE most *important pre-op medication?*

A. Carbimazole
B. Diazepam
C. Dexamethasone
D. Propranolol
E. PTU

478. A 50-year-old woman is found to have a fasting blood glucose of 9 mmol/l. BMI is 30 kg/m². She has a history of polycystic ovarian disease.

What is the SINGLE next most *appropriate management*?

A. Check creatinine prior to commencing metformin
B. Check HbAIC
C. Commence insulin
D. Commence sulfonylurea
E. Give dietary advice alone and recheck FBG in 3 months

479. A 30-year-old female who has returned from Africa 1 month ago, now complains of fever, malaise and is noted to have faintly erythematous maculopapules (rose spots) on her torso.

What is the SINGLE *investigation with the highest sensitivity*?

A. Blood culture
B. Bone marrow biopsy
C. Stool culture
D. Typhidot M test (IgG and IgM antibody test)
E. Urine culture

480. A 50-year-old man would like to have his cholesterol checked. He would like to know how long he has to 'fast' before his blood test.

What is the SINGLE *best answer*?

A. 2 hours
B. 4 hours
C. 8 hours
D. 12 hours
E. 24 hours

481. A 60-year-old woman who had undergone appendicectomy 3 weeks ago, now presents with fever and non-productive cough. Erect CXR shows air under the diaphragm. FBC shows a leukocytosis.

What is the SINGLE most *likely diagnosis*?

A. Diaphragmatic hernia
B. Perforated peptic ulcer
C. Psoas abscess
D. Subhepatic abscess
E. Subphrenic abscess

482. A 40-year-old woman complains of pain and coldness in her fingertips when it gets cold.

What is the SINGLE most *appropriate treatment*?

A. Digital sympathectomy
B. Diltiazem
C. Nifedipine
D. Prednisolone
E. Propranolol

483. A 60-year-old man with glaucoma complains of SOB and dry eyes.

What is the SINGLE most *appropriate management*?

A. Continue timolol
B. Check intra-ocular pressures
C. Change to xalatan
D. Refer urgently to ophthalmology
E. Start trial of salbutamol inhaler

484. A 70-year-old man complains of a tan brown patch on his nose with different shades of brown. He describes it as a stain on his nose that has been present for 5 years.

What is the SINGLE most *likely diagnosis*?

A. Basal cell carcinoma
B. Lentigo maligna
C. Malignant melanoma
D. Solar keratosis
E. Squamous cell carcinoma

485. A 30-year-old female with SLE now presents with a painful right red eye, tearing and photophobia. VA is diminished.

What is the SINGLE most *appropriate treatment*?

A. Acyclovir
B. Chloramphenicol drops
C. Cyclopentolate and prednisolone
D. NSAIDs
E. Sodium cromoglycate drops

486. An 11-year-old girl complains of knee pain worse when climbing up and down the stairs and running. On examination, pain is elicited over the tibial tubercle and when squatting with the knee in full flexion.

What is the SINGLE most *likely diagnosis*?

A. Chondromalacia patellae
B. Osgood-Schlatter disease
C. Patellar tendonitis
D. Patellofemoral stress syndrome
E. Quadriceps tendon avulsion

487. A 50-year-old woman had a recent ear infection and now presents with a swollen, erythematous, painful rash on her left cheek and high fever.

What is the SINGLE most *likely diagnosis*?

A. Anthrax
B. Contact dermatitis
C. Erysipelas
D. Impetigo
E. Herpes zoster

488. A 10-year-old boy presents with high fever and infected eczema on his leg. The rash has a sharply raised border and is well demarcated from the surrounding skin.

What is the SINGLE most *likely organism*?

A. Group A beta-haemolytic *Streptococcus*
B. Group B *Streptococcus*
C. Candidal organism
D. *Staphylococcus aureus*
E. *Staphylococcus epidermidis*

489. A 50-year-old inpatient has diarrhoea while on treatment for osteomyelitis.

What is the SINGLE most *likely organism*?

A. *Clostridium difficile*
B. *Clostridium perfringens*
C. *E. coli*
D. *Salmonella typhoid*
E. *Shigella*

490. A 40-year-old man with epilepsy would like to know when he can stop taking his epileptic medication?

What is the SINGLE *best answer*?

A. 1 year fit-free
B. 2 years fit-free
C. 3 years fit-free
D. 4 years fit-free
E. 5 years fit-free

491. A 50-year-old man has undergone coronary artery bypass surgery and would like to know when he can resume driving.

What is the SINGLE *best answer*?

A. 2 weeks
B. 4 weeks
C. 6 weeks
D. 2 months
E. 6 months

492. A 30-year-old woman with generalised tonic–clonic seizures requires treatment.

What is the SINGLE most *appropriate treatment*?

A. Clonazepam
B. Gabapentin
C. Phenytoin
D. Sodium valproate
E. Vigabratin

493. A 35-year-old woman presents with a discrete breast lump that persists after her next period.

What is the SINGLE most *appropriate management*?

A. Arrange mammogram
B. Arrange ultrasound
C. Non-urgent referral to breast clinic
D. Reassure that it is a fibroadenoma
E. Urgent referral to breast clinic

494. A 55-year-old man presents with hoarseness for 4 weeks. CXR is negative. He smokes 20 cigarettes a day and drinks 25 units of alcohol a week.

What is the SINGLE most *appropriate management*?

A. Prescribe penicillin V
B. Prescribe antiseptic lozenges
C. Reassure him that he has a viral infection and not to use his voice
D. Refer routinely to head and neck clinic
E. Refer urgently to head and neck clinic

495. A 50-year-old man with psoriasis complains of joint pains.

What is the SINGLE most *appropriate initial treatment*?

A. Cyclosporine
B. Diclofenac
C. Methotrexate
D. Narrow band UVB phototherapy
E. Trimovate cream

496. A 55-year-old man presents with bone pain, depression, renal stones and abdominal pain.

What is the SINGLE most *definitive treatment*?

A. Long-term steroid therapy
B. Parathyroidectomy
C. Prolonged phlebotomy
D. Radiation therapy
E. Transphenoidal hypophysectomy

497. A 40-year-old female is diagnosed with Grave's disease. She is treated but then develops a sore throat.

What is the SINGLE most *important investigation now*?

A. ESR
B. Thyroid function tests
C. Urea/ lytes
D. Ultrasound
E. White blood cell count

498. A 40-year-old man on antidepressants now presents with coma. BP is 80/50. Pupils are dilated. Reflexes are exaggerated with extensor plantar responses.

What is the SINGLE most *important treatment*?

A. IV N-acetylcysteine
B. IV flumazenil
C. IV glucagon
D. IV naloxone
E. IV sodium bicarbonate

499. A 9-month-old baby is irritable and fails to gain weight. Stools are pale and bulky.

What is the SINGLE most *definitive investigation*?

A. Barium enema
B. Endomysial antibodies
C. Full blood count and haematinics
D. Jejunal biopsy
E. Stool for reducing sugars

500. A 60-year-old smoker presents with cough and weight loss. CXR shows a solitary pulmonary nodule in the periphery.

What is the SINGLE most *appropriate investigation*?

A. Bronchoscopy and biopsy
B. FDG-PET scan
C. Percutaneous transthoracic needle biopsy
D. Sputum cytology
E. Surgical biopsy

Answers to 500 Single Best Answer Questions

1. E. Endometrial carcinoma should always be suspected as a cause for PMB. TV ultrasound should show endometrial hyperplasia, which can then be biopsied.

2. B. If you miss 2 pills in a row in the first week or 4 consecutive pills midweek, then you require emergency contraception (levonelle-2 1.5 mg stat.). Levonorgestrel is no longer recommended in two doses, i.e. 750 mcg now and 750 mcg in 12 hours.

3. A

4. E

5. B

6. A

7. E

8. E. Signs and symptoms of cauda equina syndrome.

9. B. If your index of suspicion is high, then admit to hospital for suspected malaria.

10. E. The woman is pregnant so carpal tunnel release is not an option.

11. B. Fracture of the long bone is a risk factor for fat emboli.

12. C

13. E

14. A

15. C

16. C

17. E. This boy will need nebuliser treatment with salbutamol.

18. E

19. B

20. A

21. E

22. E. This deer tick is prevalent in the New England states.

23. C. Polycystic kidney disease.

24. E

25. B. Insulation companies used to use asbestos as insulation material.

26. C

27. D. The mirena IUS is now licensed for both contraception and menorrhagia treatment.

28. E. ASCOT trial (*Lancet* Sept 2005) advocates use of amlodipine and perindopril over thiazide and beta-blocker.

29. E

30. D

31. C

32. E

33. E

34. A

35. B

36. A. This can be treated with topical Efudix.

37. C. Extradural bleed from the middle meningeal artery is often associated with a lucid interval.

38. A. Raccoon or panda eyes and haemotympanum are both seen in basilar skull fractures.

39. A

40. D. Any patient on chronic steroids must be covered by both a bisphosphonate (to protect against osteoporosis) and a PPI (lansoprazole) to protect against peptic ulcer disease else litigation is indefensible in a court of law.

41. A

42. E. Transrectal ultrasound and biopsy.

43. D. Venlafaxine and tricyclic antidepressants are cardiotoxic.

44. B. This is covered in the NICE guidelines for Eating Disorders, Jan 2004.

45. E. Case of renal colic from dehydration.

46. D

47. E. Salbutamol inhaler is indicated here.

48. C. Case of acute pulmonary oedema.

49. C

50. C. Case of stone in the common bile duct.

51. C

52. A

53. B. See NICE guideline on dyspepsia, August 2004.

54. A

55. D

56. E

57. D

58. B

59. D

60. E. Otosclerosis is an autosomal dominant disease that often presents during pregnancy.

61. C

62. B

63. C

64. E. Immersion in hot water and simple analgesia.

65. A

66. D

67. C

68. A

69. D. Annual eye tests should be offered to VDU screen users as part of occupational health.

70. B. Case of acute glaucoma. Normal IOP is between 10 and 21 mmHg.

71. B. This is a leading cause of blindness. Wet is worse than dry AMD.

72. E

73. B. The lesion is necrobiasis lipoidica seen in diabetics.

74. B. Ménière's disease results in a low-frequency sensorineural hearing loss.

75. B

76. A

77. A. Propranolol, a beta-blocker, is contraindicated in asthmatics.

78. D. Case of scabies.

79. B

80. A

81. C

82. A. Gower's manouevre described here.

83. A

84. D

85. E

86. C

87. B. If Ringer's lactate is not available, normal saline is an alternative option.

88. E. Infectious mononucleosis can cause splenic rupture so patients are advised to avoid contact sports for 6 weeks after diagnosis. Professional athletes may wish to have an ultrasound of the spleen to exclude splenic hypertrophy.

89. D. Case of enlarged adenoids. Most surgeons will carry out a T+A due to postoperative airway obstruction from tonsils.

90. B. Case of glue ear. Grommets are suggested for persistent hearing loss of 40 db.

91. D

92. A

93. E. Optic neuritis is associated with multiple sclerosis.

94. E

95. C

96. A

97. E

98. B. This is then confirmed by temporal artery biopsy. The key message is to treat with steroids to avoid blindness.

99. A

100. B. Iatrogenic injury to the parathyroid glands during thyroidectomy may result in hypocalcaemia.

101. C. Nasal vestibulitis is due to staphylococcal carriage.

102. B

103. C. Thiazides, beta-blockers and calcium channel blockers are all associated with impotence as a potential side effect.

104. C

105. A

106. A

107. C

108. D (accidental).

109. A. Incidental painless unilateral tonsillar hypertrophy must always be biopsied, i.e. tonsillectomy.

110. A

111. C

112. D

113. C

114. B. Kerr's sign of referred pain to shoulder.

115. E

116. C

117. B

118. A

119. C

120. B. Common skin finding in HIV disease.

121. E

122. C. Kaposi's sarcoma should always be suspected in a patient at risk of HIV with chronic subconjunctival haemorrhage.

123. A

124. A. Endocervical swab for chlamydia and HVS for GC, TV and thrush are recommended.

125. D

126. D

127. C

128. E

129. C

130. C

131. C. Case of intussusception.

132. D

133. A. Single word at age 1, phrases at age 2, and complete sentences at age 3 is a simple way of remembering normal speech milestones.

134. B

135. E

136. E

137. B. Septic shock. A full infection screen is recommended.

138. D

139. A. US to confirm abscess.

140. A. Case of ischaemic colitis.

141. B

142. C

143. D

144. D

145. C. Case of acromegaly. May require transphenoidal surgery.

146. C. EEG also acceptable but not gold standard.

147. E

148. C

149. A. Coeliac disease is associated with both iron and folate deficiencies.

150. A

151. D. The pupil dilates in the evening and closes off the angle. This is a case of acute angle-closure glaucoma and is an ophthalmic emergency.

152. E

153. D

154. B

155. B

156. B

157. C

158. A. ACE inhibitors are recommended for diabetics with concomitant hypertension. Check urea/lytes to ensure no renal artery stenosis.

159. C

160. D

161. A

162. C

163. D

164. A

165. E

166. E. Patients who have had mastoid surgery are often seen in the ENT clinic for microsuction of wax build-up. Wax results in a conductive hearing loss.

167. E

168. C

169. A

170. A

171. A. Subluxation of the radial head may be manipulated without analgesia.

172. C

173. A. Clavicle fracture.

174. E

175. B

176. B

177. D

178. B

179. B. Resuscitate the patient before attempting tamponade of the bleed. It is vital to have IV access established first.

180. D. Case of tension pneumothorax.

181. A

182. E. Case of renal colic. Confirm blood in urine and give IM diclofenac.

183. D

184. B. Case of ectopic pregnancy.

185. A

186. B

187. A. Fracture of the clavicle is associated with birth trauma.

188. D

189. E

190. E

191. A

192. A

193. A

194. D

195. D

196. C

197. E

198. D

199. E

200. D. Another case of PMB requiring investigation to exclude endometrial CA.

201. A

202. E

203. D

204. A

205. E

206. B

207. D

208. E

209. A. Conn's syndrome is associated with increased aldosterone production.

210. A. Case of coeliac disease.

211. C

212. D. There has been a recent alert on this class of drug potentiating suicide in children.

213. A

214. A

215. D. Lithium increases risk of hypothyroidism, so TFTs should be checked every 6 months.

216. B. The symptoms are both extrapyramidal and other side effects of antipsychotics.

217. D

218. C

219. D

220. B

221. C

222. A

223. C

224. E

225. D

226. B

227. D

228. D

229. D

230. C

231. E

232. E. Iatrogenic injury to the recurrent laryngeal nerve during thyroidectomy is a cause for litigation. Surgeons always ensure that the nerve was intact preoperatively.

233. B

234. E

235. E

236. C

237. B. D is also acceptable.

238. E

239. A

240. E. TCAs would be first-line therapy for postherpetic neuralgia but she is on digoxin, which would suggest cardiac disease. TCAs are cardiotoxic so should be avoided.

241. A. Children < 10 years old have a 90% false-negative Monospot test.

242. D

243. E. Also coined the 'morning after pill' in San Francisco.

244. A

245. A

246. B

247. D

248. D

249. C

250. B

251. D

252. A

253. C

254. E

255. D

256. E

257. D. Administer IV fluids early, as pregnant women can lose 35% of their intravascular volume before they start showing signs of hypovolaemia.

258. B. Noise-induced hearing loss shows a classic dip at 4 kHz. The patient should then have recruitment testing.

259. C

260. C

261. D

262. A

263. A

264. C

265. C

266. A

267. B. Doses given according to British National Formulary, 2005.

268. C

269. B. First kill the insect and then arrange ENT to extract.

270. A. A pea will expand on syringing. The child is uncooperative so needs to be sedated for removal under GA.

271. C

272. C

273. C. Metronidazole gel is recommended for all fungating malignancies.

274. A

275. D

276. E. Coproxamol contains dextropropoxyphene (opioid) and paracetamol. It is the dextropropoxyphene that causes lethal respiratory depression and cardiac arrhythmia. Most patients are dead before they arrive to A&E. Coproxamol has been withdrawn due to increase in suicide fatalities.

277. D

278. C

279. A

280. B. Then dextrose solution, D or E, if no response after 10 minutes.

281. C. Hyoscine crosses the BBB and causes agitation so palliative care teams now prefer glycopyrronium. However for PLAB, answer hyoscine if no glycopyrronium option as the examiners may not be current.

282. D. For genetic testing, a blood sample from a live relative with cancer is required. This woman falls into the moderate-risk category and may be referred to the breast-screening clinic (secondary care) as per NICE guidelines.

283. C

284. C

285. D

286. A

287. E

288. D

289. A. E is also acceptable. Formication is also known as the 'coke bugs'.

290. C. Although D is also acceptable.

291. B

292. C. Options A and B are diagnostic and not screening tests.

293. A

294. C. Blepharitis is treated with simple lid hygiene and is common in people with long eyelashes.

295. B

296. D

297. C

298. D

299. A

300. D

301. D

302. C

303. D

304. D

305. A. Or methylprednisolone IV.

306. A

307. C. Neuroleptic drugs may cause oculogyric crisis.

308. B. Mefenamic acid (Ponstan) is a prostaglandin synthetase inhibitor.

309. D. Fibroids are common in Afro-Carribean females and tranexamic acid is a conservative treatment of menorrhagia.

310. E

311. D

312. B

313. E

314. D

315. B

316. B. The most common site for colorectal cancer is the rectum.

317. C

318. D

319. C

320. B. ARR% = % treated group with desired outcome minus % controls with desired outcome.

321. A

322. D. Relative risk is % treated group with desired outcome divided by % controls with desired outcome.

323. A

324. C. This is to ensure that the baby does not wiggle its way under the covers down the bed.

325. C

326. D

327. C. Autosomal recessive condition.

328. C

329. B. Classic boxer's fracture.

330. B. Carrying a baby is a risk factor for this form of teno-synovitis.

331. D. Case of osteogenesis imperfecta.

332. C. Then do CT scan. Need to check the integrity of the optic nerve by checking colour vision to determine urgency of decompression.

333. D. Chronic AF with unstable MI necessitates electro-cardioversion.

334. D

335. B. Need to exclude bladder CA.

336. E

337. C

338. A

339. B

340. E

341. B. Case of gonococcal urethritis.

342. C

343. D

344. E

345. C. Community acquired pneumonia.

346. C

347. A

348. B

349. B. Pre-echo test. CHF work-up should include CXR, ECG and BNP.

350. D

351. A

352. D. SLR should elicit pain between 30 and 70 degrees. If less than this, then suspect malingering.

353. D

354. E

355. B. Epidural abscess is life threatening and requires urgent decompression.

356. B

357. E

358. C

359. E

360. C

361. E

362. C

363. C. Posterior shoulder dislocations occur with seizures and electric shocks.

364. E. One-stop rectal clinics can offer flex sigmoidoscopy for reassurance.

365. D

366. E

367. C

368. E

369. C

370. D

371. C. Gout is aggravated by thiazides.

372. B

373. C. Increasing the frequency of breastfeeds to 12 times a day will decrease BR. Phototherapy is suggested for high BR or rapidly increasing BR.

374. A

375. D. Retinal detachment (3Fs – field defect, floaters, flashers).

376. A

377. C. Cone biopsy if the lesion extends into the mucosa of the cervical canal.

378. E

379. B

380. C

381. E. Wernicke–Korsakoff due to thiamine deficiency.

382. C

383. A. Double-bubble sign signifies duodenal atresia. These scan findings suggest Down's syndrome and a second-trimester amnio should be offered. Women < 35 years old should be offered the triple test (low AFP, low oestriol and 2-fold increased hCG) and > 35 years old CVS or amnio, as the risk of a Down's baby is 1/365 in a 35-year-old and 1/30 in a 45-year-old.

384. D

385. D. Intracardiac shunt.

386. A

387. D

388. A

389. D

390. E

391. D

392. A

393. E

394. D

395. E. The Royal College of General Practitioners has published guidelines on the management of low back pain. Bedrest is not advocated.

396. D

397. D

398. E

399. A

400. B. Case of SLE.

401. B

402. D. Case of suspected splenic rupture.

403. E

404. C

405. E

406. E

407. C

408. C

409. E

410. B

411. B

412. E. Asthma is a contraindication to adenosine, else adenosine would have been the drug of choice.

413. D

414. C. Elder abuse, i.e. NAI.

415. C

416. B

417. C. Transverse temporal bone fracture on the other hand would be associated with a sensorineural hearing loss with involvement of VIII.

418. A

419. E

420. D

421. A. Age-related macular degeneration. Wet type is treated with lasers.

422. D

423. B

424. C

425. B

426. D

427. E

428. C

429. D. Dressler's syndrome is acute pericarditis post MI or CABG and is treated with ASA and NSAIDs.

430. D

431. D

432. C

433. B. Renin and aldosterone levels are both high in renal artery stenosis and both low in Cushing's disease.

434. E

435. D. Contact lens users are more prone to *Pseudomonas*-infected corneal ulcers so should be given antibiotic coverage against Gram-negative organisms.

436. A

437. E

438. B. Data from the National Statistics Office.

439. C. Syntocinon should never be administered as a bolus under any condition.

440. C

441. C

442. C. Endometriosis.

443. E. Rupture of an ovarian cyst is seen with endometriosis. Cysts may be 20 cm in size!

444. C. Mitral valve prolapse may be seen in Fragile X syndrome.

445. C

446. B

447. A. Distance squint may be a sign of myopia.

448. E

449. D

450. B. The Health Protection Agency found 23 cases of *Legionella* out of 88 spa pools inspected. The organism may be inhaled through the jets from spa pools. *Legionella* may also have been spread through air-conditioning units.

451. D

452. D

453. B

454. D. E is acceptable.

455. D

456. E

457. A

458. E

459. D. A is acceptable.

460. B. Premarin is offered if she had undergone a hysterectomy.

461. C. HELLP: Haemolytic anaemia, Elevated Liver enzymes, Low Platelets.

462. E. Depo-provera is not recommended as first-line contraception in adolescents as it has been linked with osteoporosis.

463. C. NICE guidelines for depression, Dec 2004, stipulate the need for BP and ECG prior to commencement of venlafaxine, which may now only be offered in secondary care.

464. D. Vomiting in a patient with anorexia nervosa. Laxative abuse may result in metabolic acidosis.

465. E

466. C

467. E

468. C

469. B. Blunt trauma may arise to hyphaema (blood in the anterior chamber).

470. E

471. E

472. B

473. E

474. B. Infectious mononucleosis, HSP, etc. have been linked to IgA nephropathy.

475. A

476. B. Then D if still bleeding.

477. D. Also A if not already on.

478. A

479. D. 95% sensitivity (results in 3 hours) vs bone marrow biopsy 90%, blood, urine and stool cultures 70%.

480. D

481. E. Common following perforated appendix, gastric surgery, etc.

482. C. Raynaud's phenomenon.

483. C

484. B

485. C. Uveitis.

486. B

487. C

488. A. Erysipelas.

489. A. Antibiotic-associated colitis.

490. B

491. B. www.dvla.org.uk for the latest Fitness to Drive guidelines.

492. D. Carbamazepine may also be given as a first-line antiepileptic drug.

493. E. NICE guidelines for Urgent Cancer Referrals, June, 2005.

494. E. NICE guidelines for Urgent Cancer Referrals, June, 2005.

495. B. Then C.

496. B. 85% of hyperparathyroidism cases are due to a solitary adenoma.

497. E. If the white cell count shows neutropaenia, carbimazole must be stopped immediately as this drug is associated with bone marrow suppression.

498. E. Tricyclic antidepressant poisoning is treated initially with activated charcoal if the patient is alert, IV sodium bicarbonate and IV diazepam to control seizures.

499. D. Initially one would check FBC for iron and folate deficiencies, check for endomysial antibodies (70% positive), and then the definitive diagnosis is made by biopsy.

500. C. Peripheral lesions may be approached transcutaneously. Central lesions require bronchoscopy. Open surgical biopsy is the last resort.